Chair Yoga for Seniors Over 60

Regain Self-Sufficiency, Alleviate Stiff Joints & Pain, and Live a More Joyful, Energetic Life!

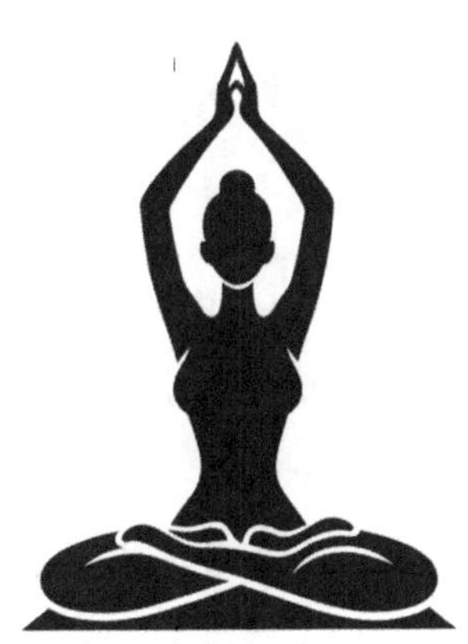

Grace Harmon

CONTENTS

Introduction

Hi, I am Grace Harmon.

I am a 68-year-old retired physical therapist and certified chair yoga instructor living in Camden, Maine. I am here to transform your life.

I have worked with countless people just like you, who want to maintain their active lifestyles as they age. They are pushing back against the narrative that the older we get, the less active and capable we become. I am here to help you change this perception by using chair yoga to facilitate physical recovery, emotional healing, and holistic well-being for those facing the challenges of aging.

I have many success stories involving chair yoga, but my favorite involves a good friend of mine who is a passionate trail runner. Daphne loves to trail run and has been running trails for years; unfortunately, she took a tumble on one of her runs and tore her anterior cruciate ligament (ACL). Although the tear was not too severe, she did require minor surgery and had a couple of months of recovery in front of her, which put her off the trails and her feet.

I was still practicing as a physical therapist, and we decided to work together to rehab her and get her back into running again. One of her main forms of rehab was chair yoga. I knew that chair yoga would be a great accessory to her other rehab protocols. I could help her rebuild her strength and flexibility with low impact and intensity, giving her body the stimulus, it needed but keeping it manageable and not too demanding.

Along with the physical stress of the injury and having to overcome it, she also battled mentally as she took time off from her favorite pastime. This is where chair yoga shone, as mindfulness created by her practice helped her develop mental resilience and positivity in what was quite a negative situation.

Like the story above with Daphne, my passion is to integrate mind, body, and spirit, while simultaneously building resilience and vitality in all my clients. I want to equip you to maintain the confidence to perform daily tasks more comfortably and safely, which in turn can enhance your self-sufficiency.

Daphne continues to integrate chair yoga into her trail running training to help keep her joints, ligaments, and muscles limber, flexible, and mobile. It became a great additional form of training that complemented her physical needs as well as the mental aspect of her sport.

Just as with Daphne, I want to help you improve your flexibility, mobility, balance, and even weight loss, if that is what you are looking for. All these skills will lead to improved physical health overall.

Additionally, as we get older, we may also begin to feel those little niggles a bit more, and we may experience chronic pain and discomfort, often due to stiff joints, muscle tightness, or back pain. I will provide you with exercises that are designed to alleviate such pains, addressing these common issues and contributing to a more comfortable and active life for you.

Chair yoga may be customized to meet you where you are in your health and wellness journey, regardless of your background or current level of fitness. Chair yoga is accessible, adaptable, and enjoyable for individuals facing various physical limitations or who are just looking for a more low-impact form of exercise.

In addition to the physical exercises, I will also provide you with guidance on the different breathing and meditation techniques that you can use to enhance mental focus, clarity, and overall well-being.

You are in for a transformative journey of both body and mind, and I am so looking forward to embarking on the journey with you. So pull up a chair and let's begin.

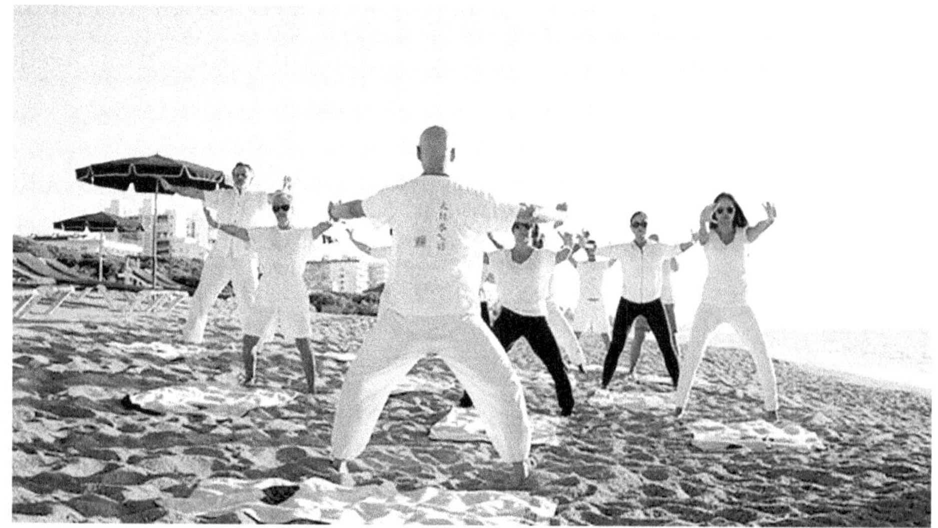

CHAPTER I

Discovering Chair Yoga

In truth, yoga doesn't take time—it gives time.

–Ganga White

The History and Evolution of Chair Yoga

Let's start from the beginning and get an idea of how modern-day yoga came to be. We will follow its path from India as it made its way to the Western World and into your hands via this book.

Tracing the Origins: A Brief History

Yoga has its roots in India, and it dates back thousands of years. Over the years, it has been modified and adapted, and we have seen a lot of changes to the traditional form of yoga. Some will argue that this means that yoga has strayed from its essence, and that may be seen as negative, but others may argue that these changes have made yoga more inclusive and popular.

Regardless of how you may feel about modern-day yoga, to garner a better understanding and appreciation for the practice, it is important to know the history.

Scholars trace the origins of yoga back 5,000 years, but some argue that it can go even further back to 10,000 years. The story follows that in India all those years ago, the first guru and yogi, Shiva, achieved enlightenment. He celebrated by alternating between dancing and sitting in complete silence.

Following the early inception of yoga, the next era was the pre-classical period, which occurred between 500-200 BCE. This occurred along with the establishment of the earliest yoga texts, known as the Upanishads and the *Bhagavad Gita*.

According to *History of Yoga: Origins to Modern Day* (2022), these two texts are the foundation on which yoga was created. The Upanishads are a collection of yoga texts that are based on Hindu philosophy, and the *Bhagavad Gita* is a poem that contains the key principles of yoga. By following these principles, one could work toward achieving enlightenment.

It was around 200 BCE-500 CE that the classical stage of yoga came about. This saw the creation of Patanjali's *Yoga Sutras*. This was another influential text, so much so that its guidance resulted in Patanjali being declared the Father of Yoga.

The eight-limbed method that the *Yoga Sutras* established for yoga practice:

Yama

This is our relationship to our environment. Within this are an additional five Yamas, which are:

Ahimsa, or non-violence
Satya, or honesty and truthfulness
Asteya, or non-stealing
Brahmacharya, or the right use of energy, marital fidelity/sexual restraint
Aparigraha, or non-greed and non-coveting
Niyama

This is our positive duty, and it consists of an additional five Niyamas:

Saucha, or cleanliness and purity of the mind and body
Santosha, which is contentment and acceptance
Tapas, which is discipline
Svadhyaya, which is study and self-reflection
Isvara Pranidhana, which is contemplation of the divine
Asana

Asana relates to the physical aspect of yoga, consisting of the poses and flows; it also refers to our posture.

Pranayama

Pranayama is the breathing technique used during practice.

Pratyahara

This relates to the withdrawal of the senses.

Dharana

Dhrana is our focused attention on a single thing.

Dhyana

This is the meditative aspect of yoga.

Samadhi

This refers to bliss or enlightenment.

As you can see, modern yoga has a strong focus on the physical pillar, but it consists of many more elements.

Post-classical yoga emerged during 500–1300 AD, and more focus emerged on asana. The change came about because yogis started to believe that enlightenment or happiness could only be attained via the physical body. Practices slowly shifted to reflect this by being designed in ways that would promote the rejuvenation of the body. This more body-centered style of yoga then went on to evolve into what we know as present-day yoga.

It was only about 300 years ago that the period of modern yoga began, when, in the 1800s, yoga masters began to travel to the West. Particularly following Swami Vivekananda's speech at the Chicago Parliament of Religions, interest in yoga has grown.

Within the modern period of yoga, we have seen the creation and growth of many different schools and styles of yoga, drawing inspiration from a variety of different sources. Now yoga is one of the leading forms of fitness and exercise, with thousands of students located across almost all the countries in the world.

Chair yoga is a more recent development; it was created as recently as 1982. According to Drake (2022), yoga practitioner Lakshmi Voelker-Binder needed to adapt her class for a student who was struggling to attempt the poses as required. Her student had arthritis and had difficulty getting down and up off the floor. Her solution? The introduction of a chair.

She took the poses and adapted them to incorporate the chair as a prop by either performing the poses seated or using the chair for balance and stability, similar to how you would use a yoga strap or block to aid you in getting into certain positions.

Lakshmi then set out to share her new methodology with others. In 2005, she opened up her teachings to others and began training teachers in her methodology. Since then, she has certified over 1,500 yoga teachers both nationally and internationally.

Understanding Chair Yoga as Adaptive Exercise

Although chair yoga was designed as an adaptive form of exercise, it can be performed by anyone. Certain groups of people gravitate to it more naturally.

Older Populations

Chair yoga has a huge following for those 65 years and older because it is so accessible, safe, and low impact. It is a great fitness method that promotes healthy aging. It has a reduced risk of falls and helps preserve balance, flexibility, functional mobility, and strength.

Those With Chronic Health Conditions

Yoga has been used as a successful tool for those with chronic disease, and the pain and symptoms related to it, to manage their ailments. Some common diseases that have shown improvement following a constant yoga practice are dementia, arthritis, and diabetes (Drake, 2022).

People With Limited Mobility

For those with mobility concerns, chair yoga makes the benefits of traditional yoga accessible. Sufferers of multiple sclerosis or those who are recovering from spinal cord injuries can benefit greatly from chair yoga.

Office Workers

Being seated and sedentary all day has many ill effects, some being fatigue, high blood pressure, and aches and pains.

Practicing yoga for a few minutes daily can help relieve lower back, neck, and shoulder pain. It can also improve stress (Drake, 2022).

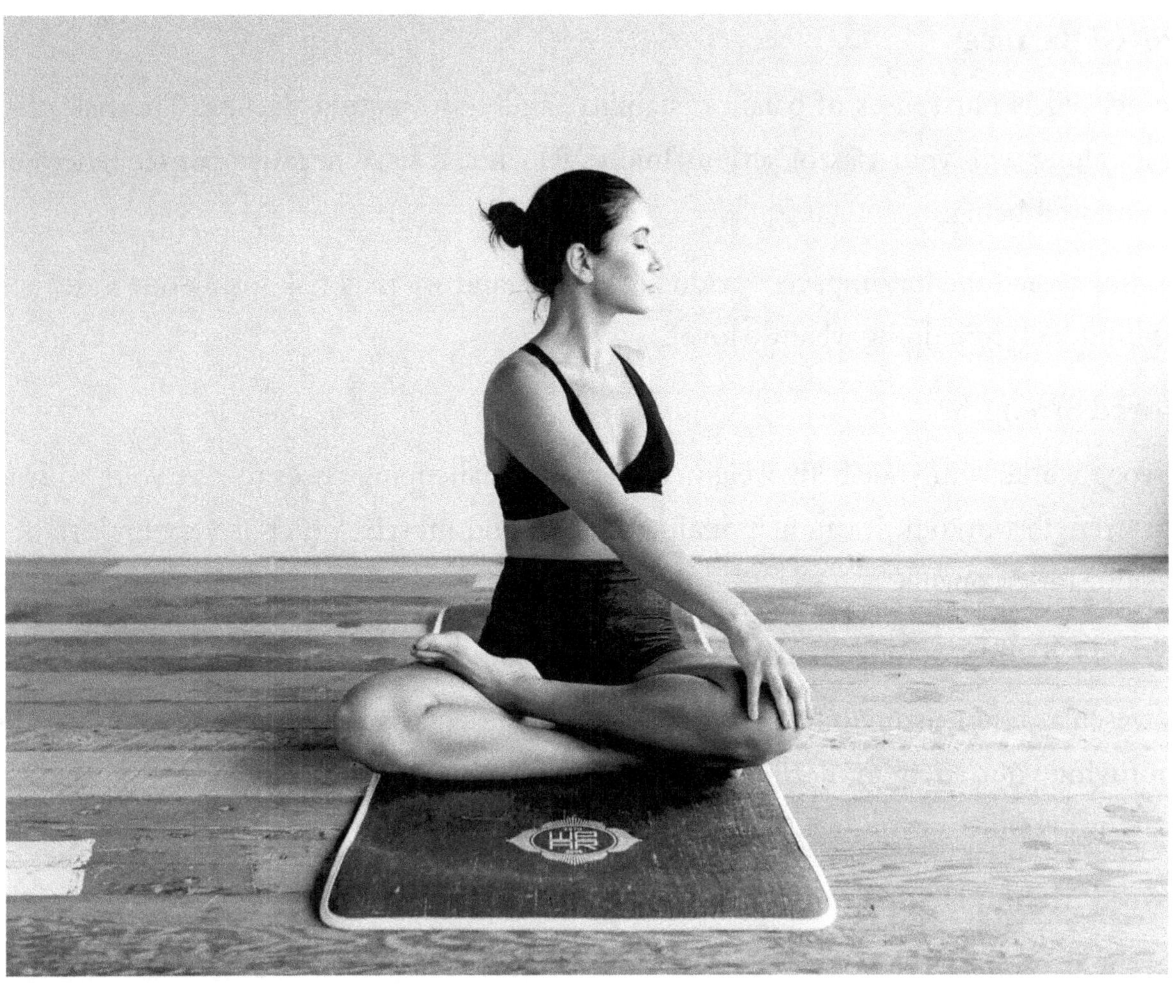

Benefits of Chair Yoga

The benefits of chair yoga range from the physical to the mental.

Increased Flexibility

There is a common misconception that you need to be able to bend like a pretzel before you start yoga if you want to be able to practice yoga effectively. This is not true.

Yoga will help you maintain and improve your flexibility. Holding each pose lets your body ease into its stretches as well as keeps it in each position for an extended amount of time, which helps improve your mobility and range of motion.

Improved Balance

As we get older, our senses of balance, stability, and coordination decline. The risk of falling increases along with your risk of serious injury, which can have negative consequences on our health and well-being.

Losing this basic function impacts our quality of life, and we may risk losing our independence and be hindered from doing what we love.

Improved Strength

Chair yoga works with your body weight, along with challenging poses to give your body a low-impact strength workout. It can help maintain and build muscle, which is very important as we get old, due to sarcopenia.

Improved Cardiovascular Health

Cardiovascular refers to anything associated with the heart. Yoga can improve your heart health. By improving your strength, flexibility, and other health markers using yoga, you can alleviate some of the pressure on your heart and decrease your risk of heart disease.

Improved Mental Health

One of the main pillars of yoga is focused on self-awareness, presence, and mindfulness. This is achieved through breathing exercises and meditation.

This focus on mental health leads to positive improvements in stress, anxiety, and low mood. Many individuals are drawn to yoga not just for its physical advantages but also for its favorable mental effects.

Improved Sleep

For those of us suffering from poor-quality sleep or having difficulty falling asleep and staying asleep, chair yoga may be the key to addressing this issue. The physical and mental effects of yoga can translate into benefits that impact your sleeping habits positively and leave you feeling more rested and rejuvenated.

Improved Pain Management

As we get older, we are more susceptible to chronic pain, be it from injuries or disease. Chair yoga generates endorphins, which are feel-good hormones released during exercise. Your body uses these hormones as its own natural painkillers.

Chair yoga is a great complementary and alternative treatment to work alongside your usual medication or therapies.

Do not take my word for this; numerous studies have been published to back up these claims. Yoga can and does make getting older easier and can counteract the process of aging (Madhivanan et al., 2021).

Success Stories: The Impact on Real Lives

At 68 years old, Sandra found that as the years passed, she became less active and perhaps indulged a bit too much in unhealthy foods.

With the natural process of aging and a decrease in physical activity, she gradually noticed her weight creeping up and her overall health declining. Not only was she physically taking strain, but she was also feeling a wide variety of different emotions. She experienced frustration at the limitations she was facing, sadness at the loss of her previous agility, and a sense of vulnerability as her body didn't respond the way it used to.

One day she had a mishap that led to her falling and breaking her ankle. Sandra misjudged a step and lost her balance, causing her to trip and fall awkwardly, which resulted in a fracture.

It was a painful and unexpected event that prompted her to focus on her health and well-being. She was determined to improve her health and regain some of the mobility and strength she had lost. It was a challenging and reflective time for her.

She discovered chair yoga through a recommendation from a friend who knew about her situation and thought it would be beneficial for her. The classes were conducted in a gentle and supportive manner, with the instructor guiding her through modified yoga poses that could be done comfortably while seated on a chair or using it for support.

Physically, she initially felt a bit hesitant but soon realized the benefits of chair yoga. Mentally, the practice brought her a sense of calmness and inner peace, allowing her to focus on the present moment and let go of any stress or worries.

Chair yoga played a crucial role in her rehabilitation from her ankle injury. It helped her improve her flexibility, balance, and overall strength gradually without putting too much strain on her recovering body. The gentle movements and mindful breathing techniques in chair yoga contributed to her healing process and also enhanced her physical and mental well-being during the recovery period.

Initially, she continued to be constantly worried about falling again, especially with the fragility of her ankle post-injury. However, as she continued practicing chair yoga and felt the improvements in strength, stability, and balance, her confidence started to grow. The supportive environment of the classes and the gradual progress she made in each session boosted her confidence and helped alleviate some of her fear of falling.

With regular practice of chair yoga and adopting a healthier lifestyle, Sandra noticed gradual weight loss over time. The combination of mindful movement, breathing exercises, and the positive impact on her overall well-being from chair yoga played a significant role in her weight management and physical fitness.

Aside from weight loss and improved physical strength, practicing chair yoga regularly brought various other benefits. She noticed increased flexibility, reduced joint stiffness, better posture, and enhanced concentration and mental clarity. Additionally, the relaxation techniques in chair yoga helped her manage stress more effectively and promoted a sense of inner peace and well-being. Overall, chair yoga became a valuable tool in her journey toward better health and wellness.

And it can be yours as well! Now that you have the history behind chair yoga, we can begin to take the practical steps to set up your yoga practice.

The following chapter will provide you with the tools to create an environment for you to practice in.

Key Takeaways

- With roots in India, yoga has a long and illustrious history that has seen it grow from a local practice to a worldwide phenomenon that is respected by many different cultures.

- The Upanishads, the *Bhagavad Gita,* and *Patanjali's Yoga Sutras* were among the fundamental books introduced throughout the classical period of yoga, helping to shape the conceptual foundations of the practice.

- Chair yoga, a more recent development in the yoga landscape, offers a modified and accessible form of exercise suitable for diverse populations, including older individuals, those with chronic health conditions, and office workers.

- The benefits of chair yoga encompass physical aspects such as increased flexibility, improved balance, strength building, and cardiovascular health, as well as mental health benefits like stress reduction, better sleep quality, and pain management.

- Real-life narratives exemplify the transformative impact of chair yoga on individuals' physical rehabilitation, weight management, and overall well-being, underscoring its value as a holistic approach to health improvement.

CHAPTER 2

Preparing for Your Chair Yoga Journey

One of the benefits of chair yoga and yoga in particular is that you do not require any special equipment. All you require is a mat and a chair.

Should you wish to set up a dedicated yoga space and invest in various props and tools, this chapter will guide you in doing so.

Setting the Scene for Safety and Comfort

Two important elements of your practice are ensuring you are safe and that you are comfortable.

The first thing you should do when it comes to safety is to talk to your healthcare provider and get the all-clear to exercise. Once you have been approved, the fun can begin.

Choosing the Right Chair for Stability and Support

The chair is in the spotlight when it comes to chair yoga, but you do not need a fancy or specific chair designed especially for chair yoga. There are a few basic requirements, but almost any chair that you have at home will work.

Depending on the chair, you may be slightly limited with some poses and may need to make additional modifications, but there are so many different variations of poses that you can do that allow you to adapt to what you have to work with.

If you do want to invest in a chair, several companies create chairs specifically for chair yoga, and a quick internet search can bring a few of these up for you.

Regardless of the chair you use, here are some useful points to consider when selecting a chair:

- the type of poses you will be practicing

- the style of chair

- the height of the backrest

- the height of the chair

- armrests

- wheels

The Standard Chair

A kitchen chair or office chair would be the go-to that most people use when beginning their practice. These are usually a standard height and will have the right dimensions for most people.

Backless Chair

A backless chair allows more freedom for movement and may make more poses accessible, but with that comes a potential loss of stability. Additionally, most common chairs are not backless, so you may need to look around to find one.

Balance Ball Chair

Balance ball chairs have risen in popularity over the years, and many people who spend a large amount of time sitting use them as alternatives to the standard desk chair. They claim to provide a way to work on your core, stability, and balance and provide a healthier alternative when sitting for a prolonged period.

These chairs usually have wheels, and as with all chairs with wheels, these can prove to be a safety hazard if not locked in position. So please ensure that they are secure.

Office Chair

Office chairs are commonly used for chair yoga. They usually have backrests, armrests, and wheels. Armrests may require you to modify some poses, and if the chair has wheels, they need to be lockable as well to ensure stability and safety.

Other Equipment

Aside from your chair, which many of you have already, there are several other props you could use that will aid your practice. Props are handy tools if you need help with your balance and stability or have flexibility and mobility limitations. They can also help deepen your stretches. It is important to remember that props aren't a measure of ability but a tool to individualize your practice.

You may find that there are several items that you can find in your home already that can be used instead of purchasing any of these.

Yoga Mat

A yoga mat can be used for any of your floor exercises and will also provide a secure surface to place your chair on, which can prevent it from slipping.

Blocks

Blocks are used to correct your alignment during asanas. They are made from wood, cork, or foam and come in various sizes and weights.

Blocks can help reduce the range of movement; for example, if you are having difficulty reaching the floor, the block will be used as your point of contact. They are very versatile and can also be used to create support and balance.

Books are a good alternative to blocks if you do not want to purchase them before trying them out.

Pillows and Bolsters

Pillows and bolsters offer the same benefits as blocks but provide more comfort. They can be used behind your head, behind your back, or for kneeling and sitting on when needed to adjust and get into better positions.

If you have a cushion, rolled-up blanket, or small pillow, you can use it instead of purchasing specific yoga ones.

Straps

Straps also reduce the range of motion should you have mobility or flexibility difficulty; they can also be used to increase your stretches. Straps come in a variety of different lengths and materials.

A belt or long strip of fabric can be a great substitute for a strap.

Dressing for Success: Appropriate Attire for Chair Yoga

There is no specific way to dress for yoga except to choose comfortable items. Here are some guidelines when choosing your yoga clothes for your practice.

Comfort

Stick to clothing that is comfortable. Remember that you will be stretching, bending over, inverted, sitting, and standing, so you need to factor in these movements. All this range of motion and movement requires that your clothes be quite flexible and stretch to accommodate the different positions.

Make sure that your clothing fits well and isn't too tight or too loose. Oversized clothing can get in your way when you are performing certain poses and distract you during your practice.

Simplistic

Pick simple items of clothing without embellishments such as ties, strings, zippers, or buttons. A basic t-shirt, shorts, or leggings are great basics to have to work in.

Cool

Opt for clothing that is breathable and will keep you cool. Choose clothing items that are made from cotton and avoid nylon or polyester. You can also get workout clothing that is made of moisture-wicking material that will keep your temperature comfortable.

Creating the Perfect Environment

If you are lucky enough to be able to set up a dedicated space for your yoga practice, I highly suggest that you do so. It does not need to be very elaborate or take up a lot of space, but the benefits of having your area to practice are well worth it.

Whether you have a tiny corner in your living or bedroom or a whole room to dedicate to it, there are many ways that you can create a place filled with serenity and peace.

Select Your Space

You do not need a lot of space for your yoga practice, nor do you need a dedicated space, although it would be preferable.

Whatever your circumstances, whether you use a corner of your room or have a room itself, the area must be a place that brings you peace, creates a calm atmosphere, and lets you let go of stress and anxiety.

It should be a space that allows you to easily realign back to your surroundings and yourself.

You should also declutter your yoga space, not only for safety reasons but also because clutter can lead to scattered thoughts. Stick to items that you need and bring you harmony during your practice and clear out all the rest.

Create a Beautiful Environment

A lot can be done with lighting, decor, and paint. Working with these elements to design your space can make a wonderful difference to your yoga area. Work with as much natural light as you can; natural light boosts serotonin levels.

If you are limited and cannot use natural light, you can use light therapy lamps. These lamps work with your sleep and wake cycle and encourage your body to release melatonin and serotonin. These lamps are very versatile, and the colors themselves can be adjusted depending on your needs.

Along with your lighting, the color of your space can also impact your mood and create a peaceful and calming ambiance. Choose natural earth tones like green, brown, and blue to promote feelings of calmness and relaxation, as opposed to colors such as red and yellow.

If your space allows for it, add mirrors to help you focus on your position and alignment. They can help you progress and work on your postures and asanas and allow you to practice while avoiding potential injuries.

Mirrors also provide a beautiful aesthetic and make small areas feel more open and spacious.

Plants and other natural elements can bring some life into your space and help you connect with your environment and the natural world. Sounds and scents will also add to your atmosphere. Relaxing music can help you focus and bring yourself inward, as it drowns out the external noises. Essential oil diffusers and candles allow your sense of smell to be involved in your practice, and you can find them in many calming aromas such as sage and lavender.

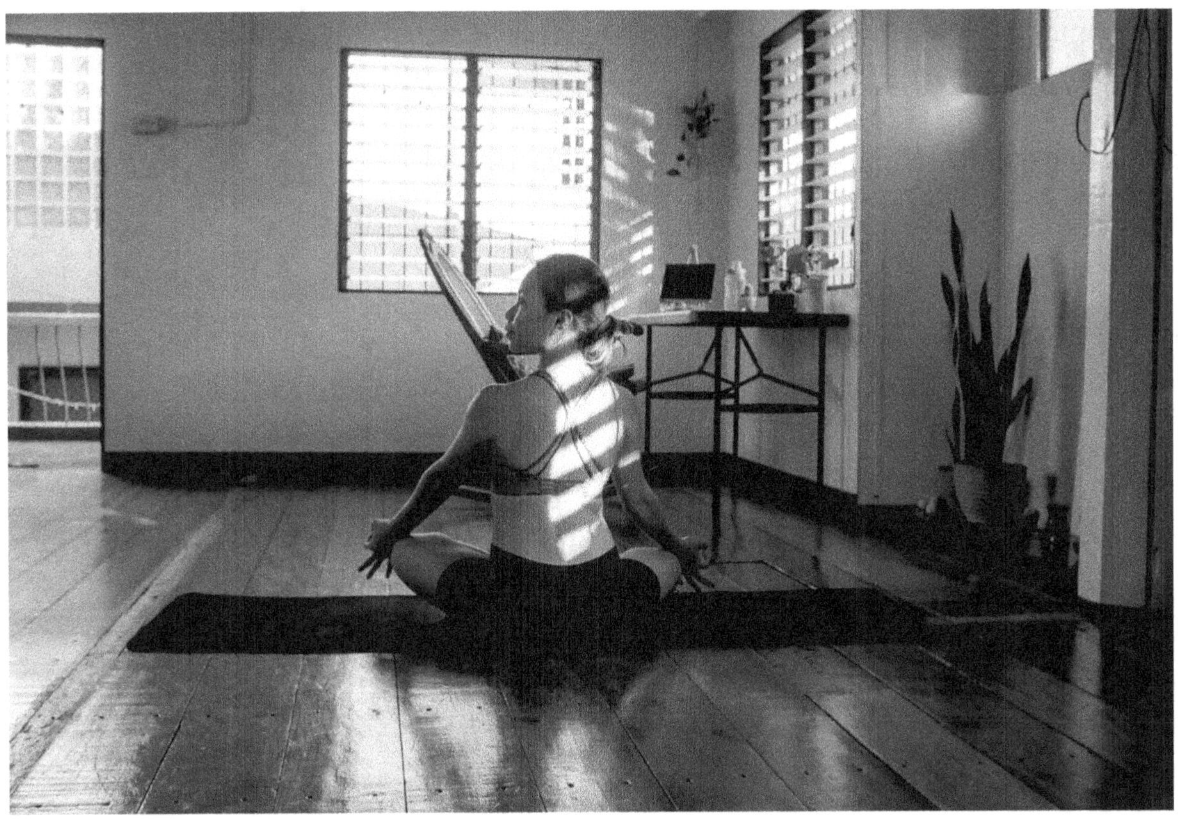

Preparing the Mind for Chair Yoga

The hardest part of anything new is just starting. Taking the leap from inaction to action, especially when it comes to something new and unfamiliar, is more about convincing the mind than anything else.

The first thing to acknowledge is that you are a beginner, and you should not be afraid of being a beginner. We all have to start somewhere. Do not be scared to get things wrong, have difficulty getting into poses and flows, being unfit or not flexible enough—those will all come in time. All you need to do is get onto the chair!

Breathing Techniques for Relaxation and Focus

Meditation and mindfulness are important pillars of yoga. The strengthening and training of the mind is on par with the importance of strengthening and training the body. Although breathing work is ingrained within yoga itself and the poses and flows, I love to add additional breathwork to my sessions either before or after.

Here are some breathing techniques you can play around with. You can use these as part of your practice or independently.

Diaphragmatic Breathing

1. Start your practice by sitting or lying in a comfortable position on your mat or your chair.
2. If you are lying on your back, keep your head cushioned and your knees slightly bent.
3. Place your left hand on your upper chest and your right hand on your abdomen, below your rib cage, so that you can feel your diaphragm moving effortlessly.
4. Breathe in slowly through your nose, as you feel your belly press into your hand.
5. Keep your other hand as still as possible.
6. Keeping your upper hand motionless, contract your abdominal muscles and release the breath via pursed lips.
7. Repeat for as many breath cycles as needed.
8. Once you are comfortable with this, you can incorporate it into your daily activities.

Pursed Lip Breathing

1. Start your practice by sitting upright in your chair and relaxing your neck and shoulders.
2. Keep your mouth closed while breathing in slowly through your nose for two counts.
3. Pucker or purse your lips as though you are going to whistle.
4. Breathe out slowly by gently blowing air through your pursed lips for a count of four.

Breath Focus Technique

1. Start your practice by sitting or lying in a comfortable position on your mat or your chair.
2. Begin to focus and bring awareness to your breath without trying to alter it and change your rhythm of breathing.
3. Switch between normal and deep breaths a few times and pay attention to any differences between the two. Notice how your abdomen expands when you are breathing in.
4. Pay attention to how shallow breathing feels compared to deep breathing.
5. Keep focusing on and practicing your deep breathing for a few minutes.
6. Put your left hand below your belly button, and keep your belly relaxed. Observe how it rises and falls with each inhalation and exhalation.

7. As you breathe out, let out a loud sigh.

8. As you begin your breath focus practice, combine this deep and focused breathing with imagery. Pick a word or phrase that supports relaxation and calm.

9. Imagine that the air that you breathe in is providing you with waves of peace and calm as it moves through your body. You can tell yourself as you breathe that you are "inhaling peace and calm."

10. Imagine the air you breathe out washing away tension and anxiety. You can tell yourself as you breathe out that you are "exhaling tension and anxiety."

Alternate Nostril Breathing

1. Start your practice by sitting upright in your chair and relaxing your neck and shoulders.

2. Raise your right hand to your nose, extending your other fingers while pressing your middle and index fingers into your palm.

3. Using your right thumb, softly shut your right nostril after exhaling.

4. Using your right pinky and ring fingers, shut your left nostril after taking a breath through it.

5. Release your thumb and exhale through your right nostril.

6. Inhale through your right nostril and then close this nostril.

7. In order to exhale from your left nostril, release your fingers.

8. This is one cycle.

9. Continue this breathing pattern for up to five minutes.

10. Finish your session with an exhale on the left side.

Humming Bee Breath

1. Start your practice by sitting upright in your chair and relaxing your neck and shoulders.

2. Shut your eyes and let your face relax.

3. Place your pointer fingers on the cartilage that partially covers your ear canal.

4. Breathe in and gently press your fingers into the cartilage as you begin to breathe out.

5. Begin to make a humming noise, but keep your mouth closed as you do so.

6. Continue for as long as you are comfortable.

Equal Breathing

1. Start your practice by sitting upright in your chair and relaxing your neck and shoulders.

2. Inhale and exhale through your nose.

3. As you breathe in and breathe out, keep count and make sure that they are even in duration. Or you could choose a mantra or word that you could repeat during each breath.

4. Once you get comfortable with that breathing sequence, you can add a slight pause after each inhale and exhale.

5. Continue this breathing sequence for five minutes.

Setting Your Intentions

Remember that yoga means the union of mind and body, so while we are focusing on the physical, we also need to pay attention to the mental side of our practice. This is easy to do when we set intentions.

By setting an intention, we choose what we want to focus on for our sessions, which brings clarity and focus and can help us achieve better mindfulness and presence.

Setting intentions also allows for introspection and the chance for you to really develop your relationship with yourself. When setting intentions, you are required to look at your values and what is important to you. This helps you recognize your core beliefs and the traits that you would like to cultivate within yourself.

This of course lays a great foundation for mental and emotional transformation and growth.

Goals vs. Intentions

Goals are different from intentions in that they are outcome-based and focus on the external result instead of an internal transformation. Goals are also more specific and are measurable, with outcomes that are not usually focused on values or purposes. For example, a goal could be to lose weight, which is fueled by a desire to look a certain way. An intention would be to build up your self-confidence and self-love to be able to accept and love your body as it is.

Intentions help you align your actions to your values, which creates a deeper sense of motivation; this can make it easier to reach your goals.

How to Set Intentions

1. Identify your values and take some time to reflect on what qualities and traits you want to embody and work on in your life.

2. Simplify your intentions and keep them uncomplicated. The simpler they are, the easier they are to focus on. Choose a single word or mantra that summarizes the value you want to work on, such as gratitude, peace, compassion, or confidence.

3. Personalize your intention so that it resonates and is meaningful to you. It needs to be connected to you on a deep level so that you are more likely to successfully stick to it.

4. Once you have set your intention, incorporate it into your practice. As you progress through your flows and poses, pay attention to your intention and allow it to direct your movements as you gently repeat it to yourself.

5. When you have done your session, take some time to check in with yourself and be aware of how your activity made you feel.

6. Finally, reflect on your progress and gauge how your intentions are manifesting in your daily life. Are you making progress with your self-awareness and growth?

Some examples of intentions are:

- gratitude
- compassion
- acceptance
- patience
- peace
- strength

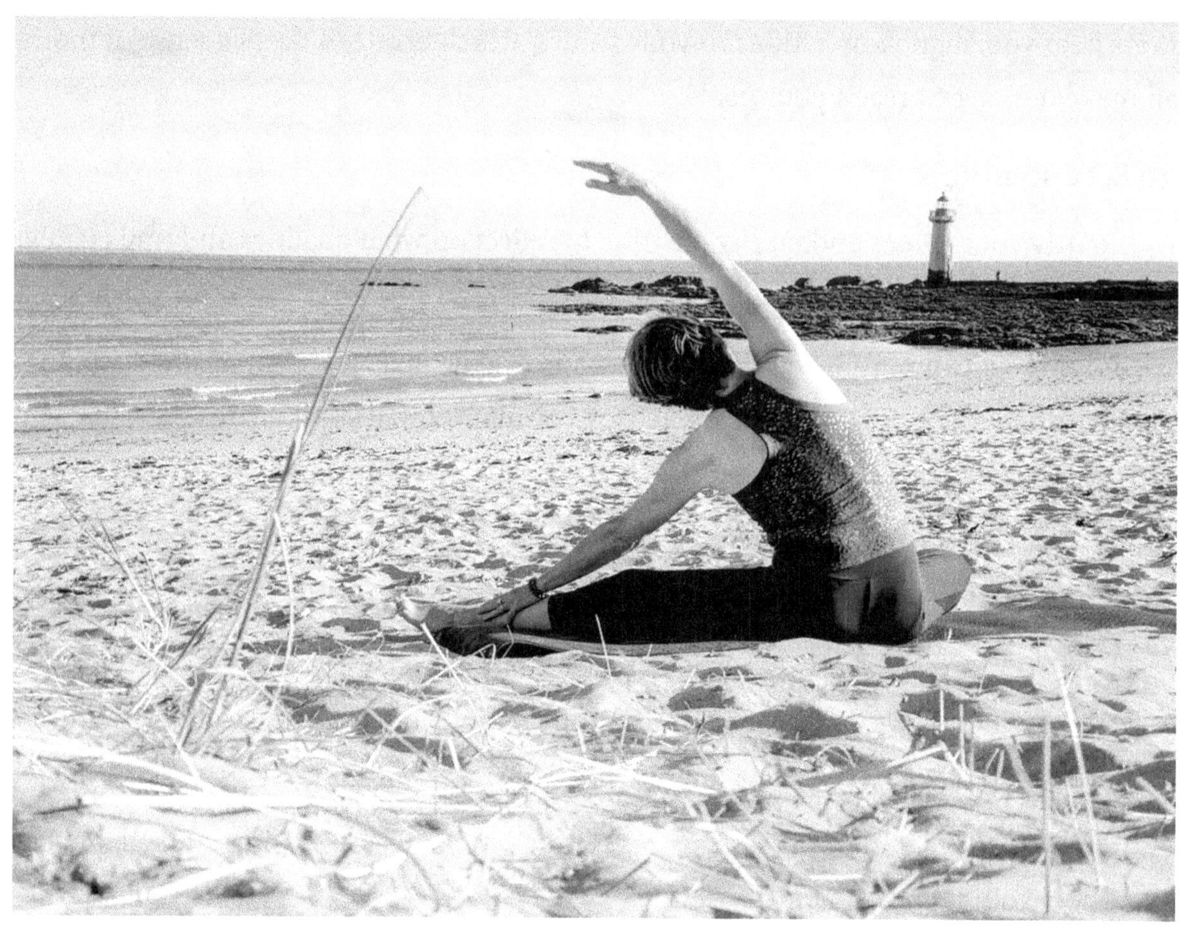

Recognizing Personal Boundaries

There will be instances where a pose or flow may be challenging, and you will need to assess whether you should persevere with the challenge or back off and adapt the pose. This is where you need to listen to the advice of your healthcare practitioner as well as your body.

While we may feel discomfort, we do not want to feel pain, especially when it may be in areas where we have previously had or currently have an injury.

We may even have days when things are off and our bodies do not want to cooperate; we may be tired, stiff, or sore. Again, you need to listen to your body and navigate around it in these instances. Take the day off, change your practice, and modify as needed to ensure you are meeting yourself where you are.

Warming Up for Chair Yoga

Although you perform chair yoga seated, do not be deceived into thinking it is an "easy" activity. It should be considered a physically challenging endeavor, and like any other physical activity, you need to warm up and cool down appropriately.

Warm-ups prepare your body for the activity it is going to perform. They elevate your heart rate and prime your cardiovascular system for the extra strain it may be about to take on. Additional benefits include increasing blood flow around the body, including the muscles, tendons, and joints, raising the body temperature, and increasing oxygen intake. These all reduce the risk of injury.

When it comes to yoga-specific warm-ups, most practices begin with the Sun Salutations; these can be used as a warm-up along with other basic stretch flows.

Seated Sun Salutations

1. Start your practice by sitting upright in your chair and relaxing your neck and shoulders. Position your feet so that they are flat on the floor and hip-width apart.

2. As you take a deep breath, lift your arms over your head and reach toward the ceiling. Ensure that your shoulders remain relaxed.

3. Breathe out and bring your palms together in a prayer position in front of your chest.

4. Breathe in and raise your arms overhead again, stretching upward.

5. Breathe out, twist your upper body to the right, and place your left hand on your right knee and your right hand on the back of the chair.

6. Breathe in and come back to the center with your arms raised.

7. Breathe out and twist your torso to the left, placing your right hand on your left knee and your left hand on the back of the chair.

8. Breathe in and come back to the center with arms raised.

9. Breathe out and lower your arms back down by your sides.

10. Repeat this flow one or more additional times.

We will go through more specific warm-ups in the next chapter.

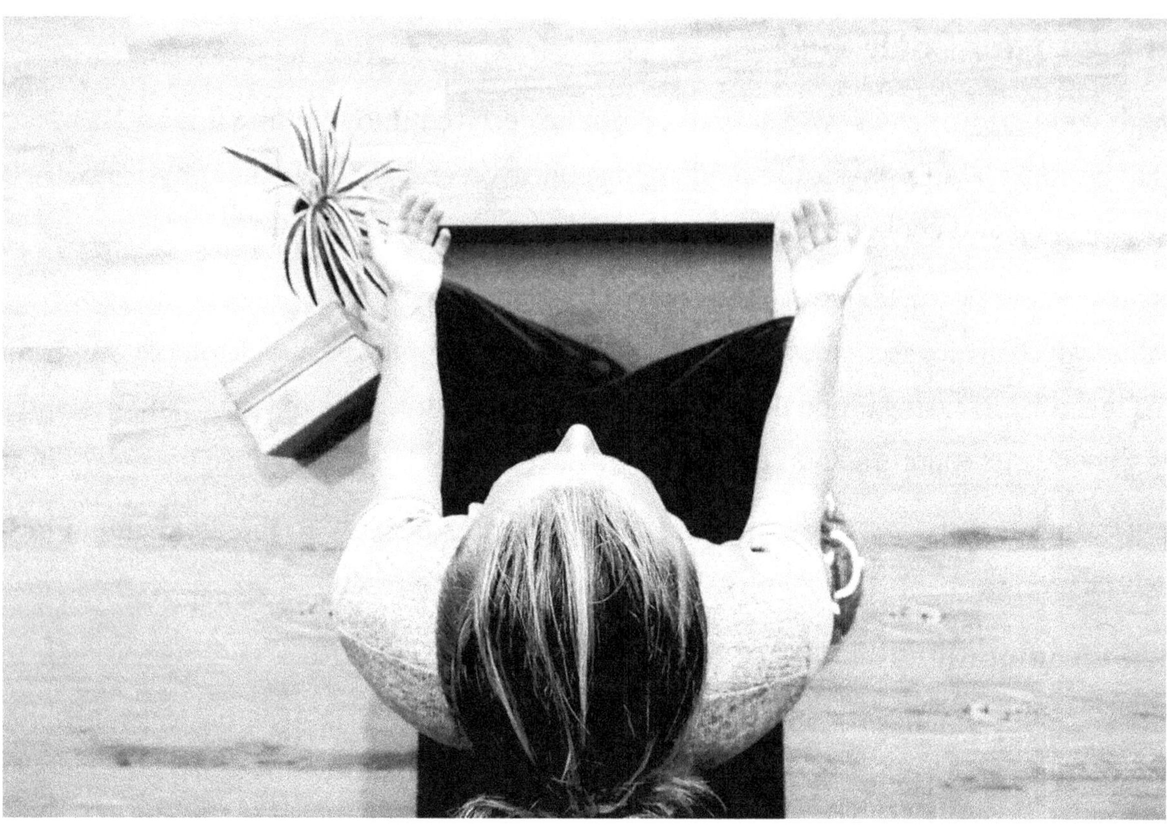

Key Takeaways

- Chair yoga requires minimal equipment, with a simple setup of a mat and a chair being sufficient to begin the practice.

- Safety and comfort are paramount, requiring individuals to seek clearance from their healthcare provider before engaging in chair yoga.

- Various chair options, including kitchen chairs and balance ball chairs, offer different levels of stability and support for chair yoga practice.

- Using props such as blocks, pillows, straps, and yoga mats can aid in enhancing balance, stability, and flexibility during chair yoga sessions.

- Dressing in comfortable, breathable clothing and creating an optimal yoga environment with calming elements can enhance the overall chair yoga experience.

- Setting intentions before practice sessions helps in focusing the mind and aligning actions with personal values for mental and emotional growth.

- Incorporating breathing techniques like diaphragmatic breathing and breath focus techniques can promote relaxation and mindfulness during chair yoga sessions.

- Warming up before chair yoga is essential in preparing the body for physical activity, reducing the risk of injuries, and incorporating practices like Sun Salutations and specific warm-up routines.

CHAPTER 3

Gentle Start – Warm-Up Routines

We touched briefly on the benefits of warm-up routines in the previous chapter. A good warm-up sets the tone for your practice.

We will be going through some basic stretches and movements that you put together to create a great warm-up sequence. We will also provide a template you can use to create your own flows.

Warm-Up Exercises

You can select any warm-up movement that relates to what you are doing during your flow. Pick one or two that you feel will warm you up sufficiently. Remember, the key is to gently move.

Neck Rolls

1. Start your practice by sitting upright in your chair and relaxing your neck and shoulders. Your feet should be flat on the floor, about hip-width apart, with your knees in line with your ankles. Your hands can be resting on your thighs.

2. Gently bring your right ear to your right shoulder, and rotate your head in a clockwise direction.

3. Rotate for as many repetitions as required.

4. Relax and switch directions.

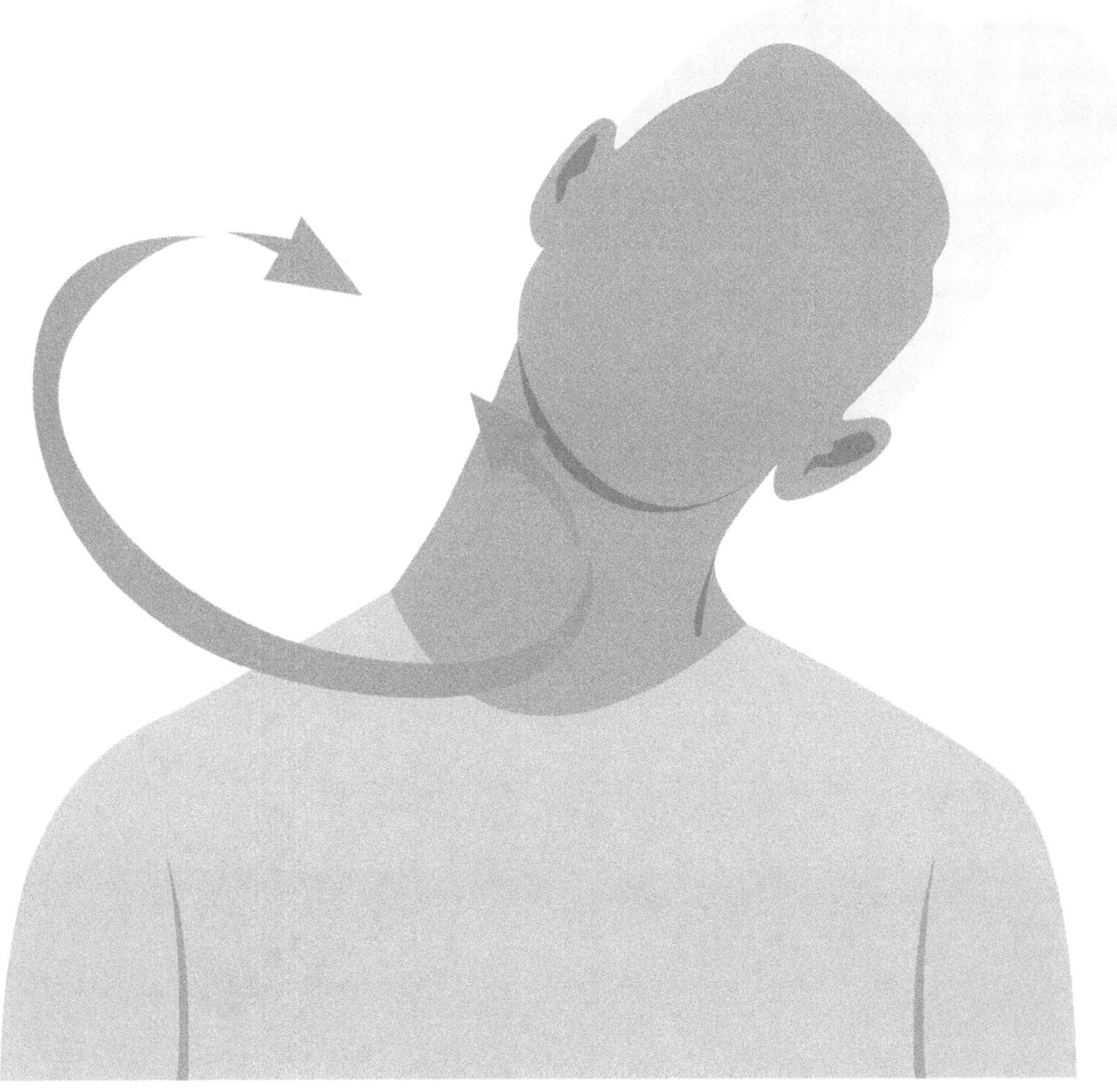

Wrist Rotations

1. Start your practice by sitting upright in your chair and relaxing your neck and shoulders. Your feet should be flat on the floor, about hip-width apart, with your knees in line with your ankles. Your hands can be resting on your thighs.

2. Raise your arms straight in front of you at shoulder height. Create two fists with your hands.

3. Slowly begin rotating your fists, from your wrists, in circular motions toward one another.

4. Repeat for 10-15 repetitions.

5. Relax and repeat in the other direction.

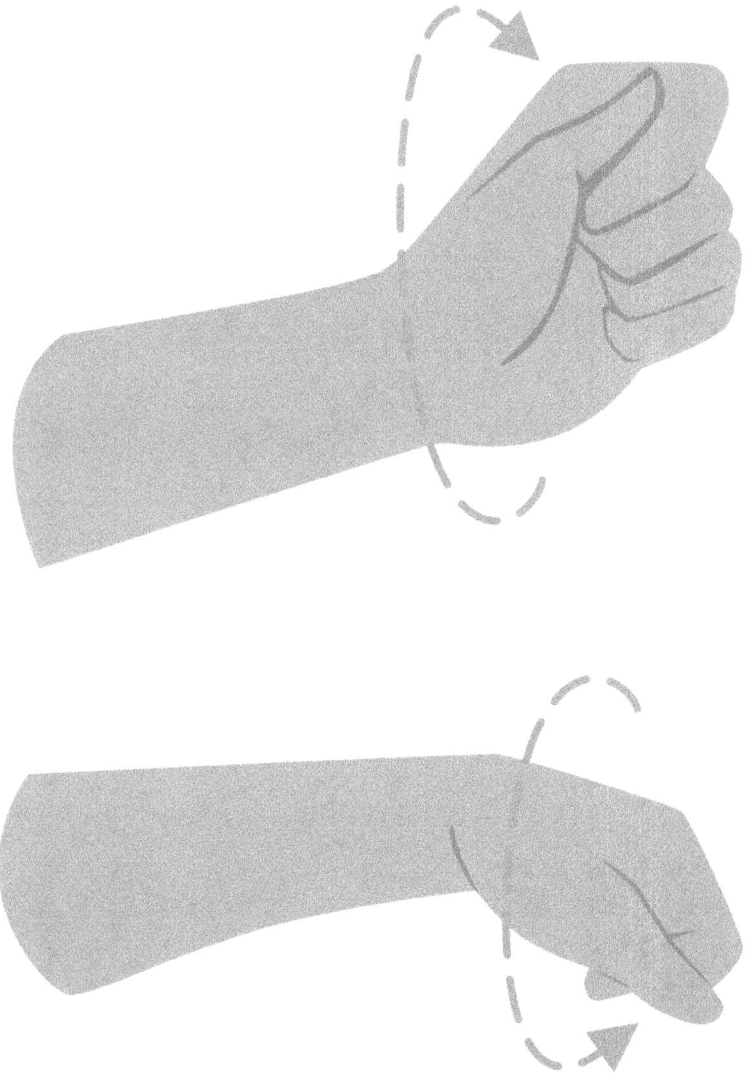

Arm Circles

1. Start your practice by sitting upright in your chair and relaxing your neck and shoulders. Your feet should be flat on the floor, about hip-width apart, with your knees in line with your ankles. Your hands can be resting on your thighs.

2. Raise your arms out to your sides in line with your shoulders.

3. Keeping your arms straight and moving from your shoulders, gently rotate your arms forward.

4. Start with small circles, and as you progress, let them get bigger.

5. Repeat for 10-15 repetitions.

6. Relax and repeat in the other direction.

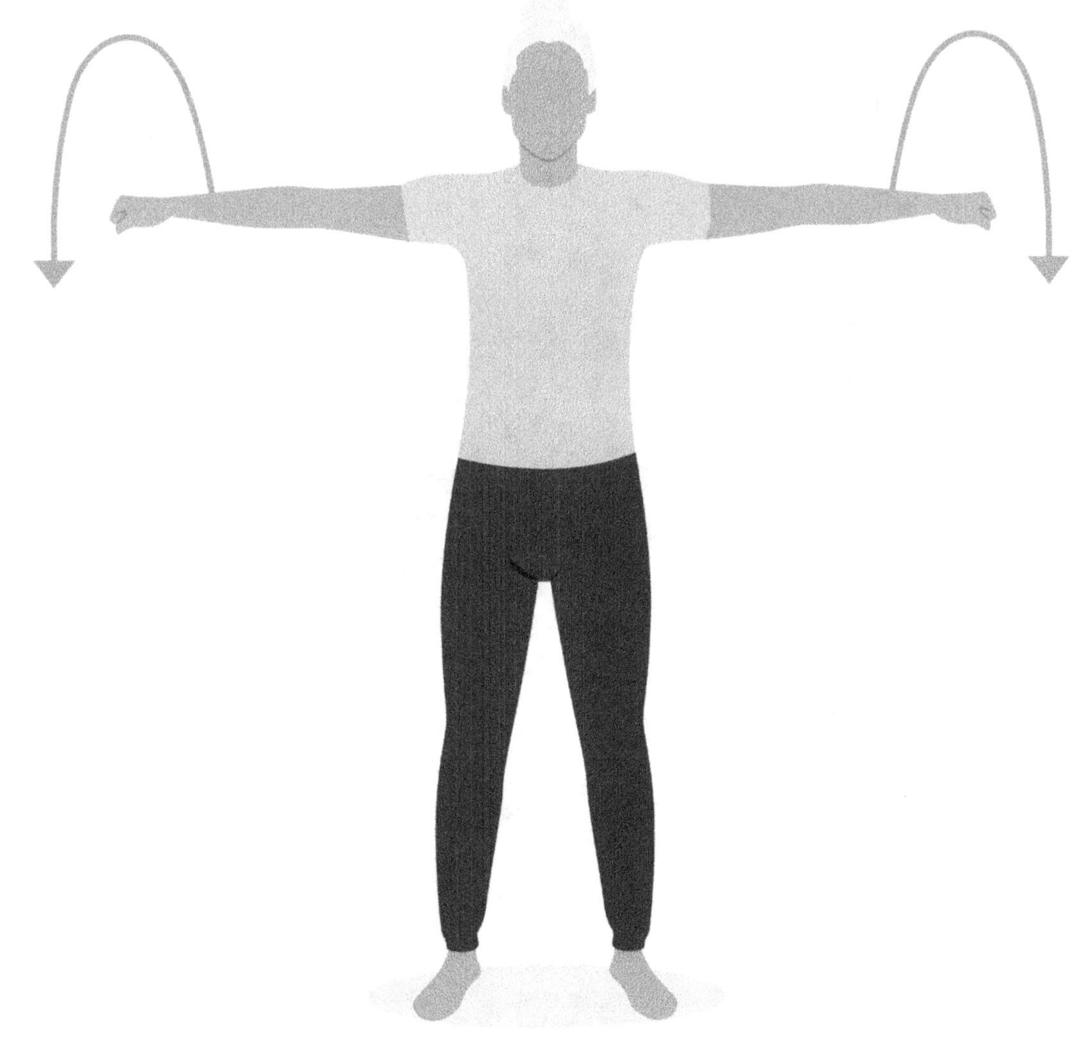

Hip Flexions

1. Start your practice by sitting upright in your chair and relaxing your neck and shoulders. Your feet should be flat on the floor, about hip-width apart, with your knees in line with your ankles. Your hands can be resting on your thighs.

2. Lift your left leg, keeping your knee bent.

3. Hold for one breath and gently lower it back to the ground.

4. Repeat for as many reps as needed.

5. Swap sides and repeat.

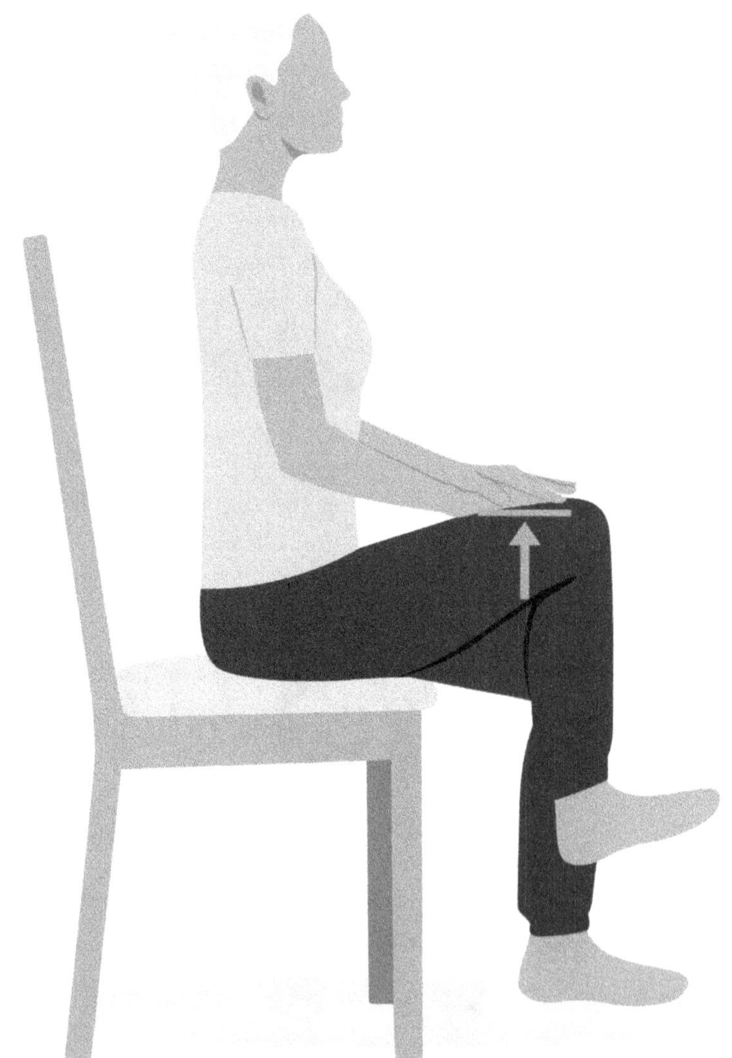

Seated Toe Touches

1. Start your practice by sitting upright in your chair and relaxing your neck and shoulders. Your feet should be flat on the floor, about hip-width apart, with your knees in line with your ankles. Your hands can be resting on your thighs.

2. Place your feet slightly out before you and your hands on your thighs.

3. Slowly slide your hands down your legs until you reach your feet.

4. Hold for as long as needed.

5. Slide your hands back up to your thighs.

6. Repeat.

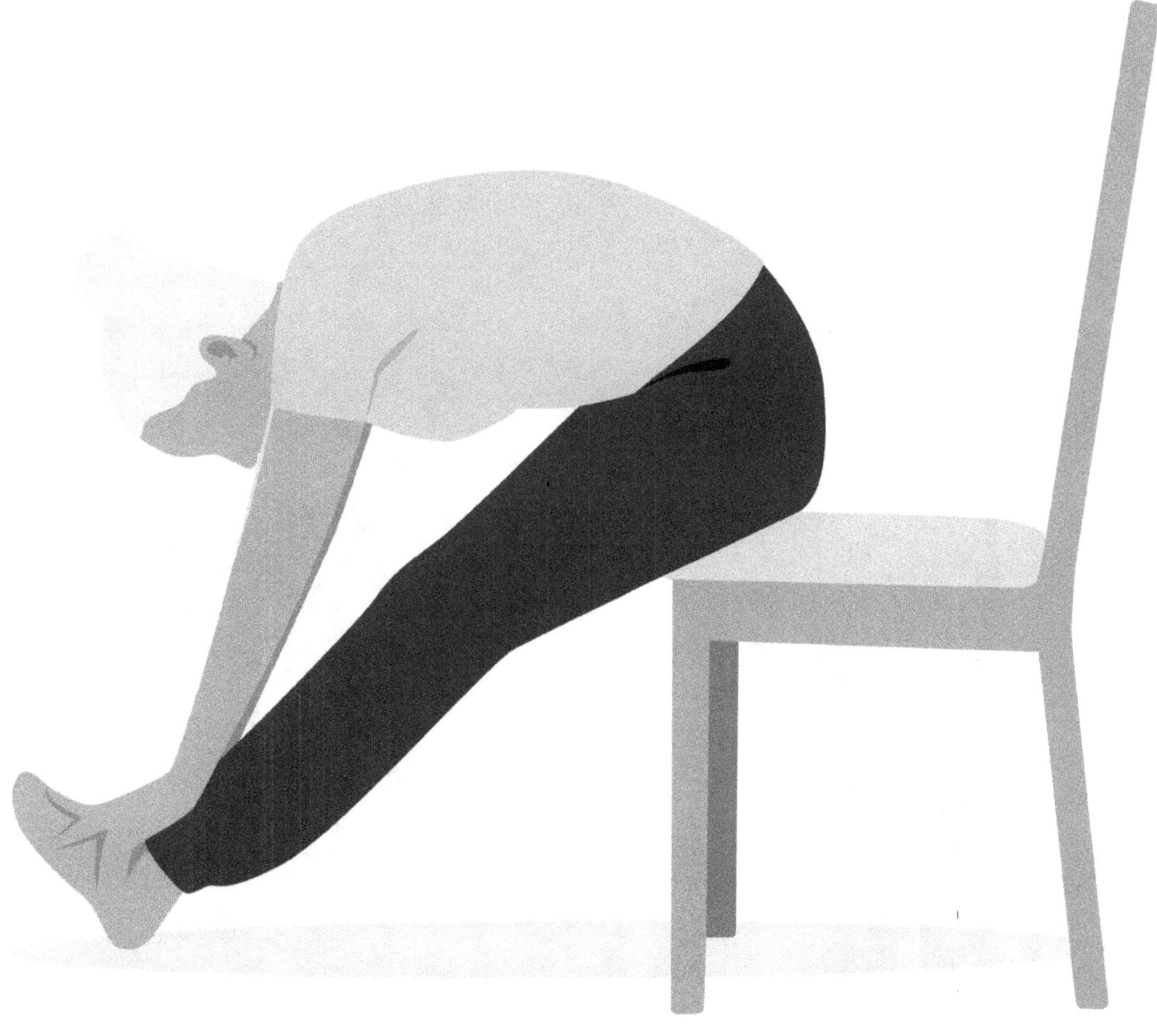

Side Bends

1. Start your practice by sitting upright in your chair and relaxing your neck and shoulders. Your feet should be flat on the floor, about hip-width apart, with your knees in line with your ankles. Your hands can be resting on your thighs.

2. Let your right arm hang beside you and place your left hand over your head.

3. Slowly lean toward your right; you should feel a stretch in your left side as you do so.

4. Hold for as long as needed.

5. Release and return to the center.

6. Swap sides and repeat.

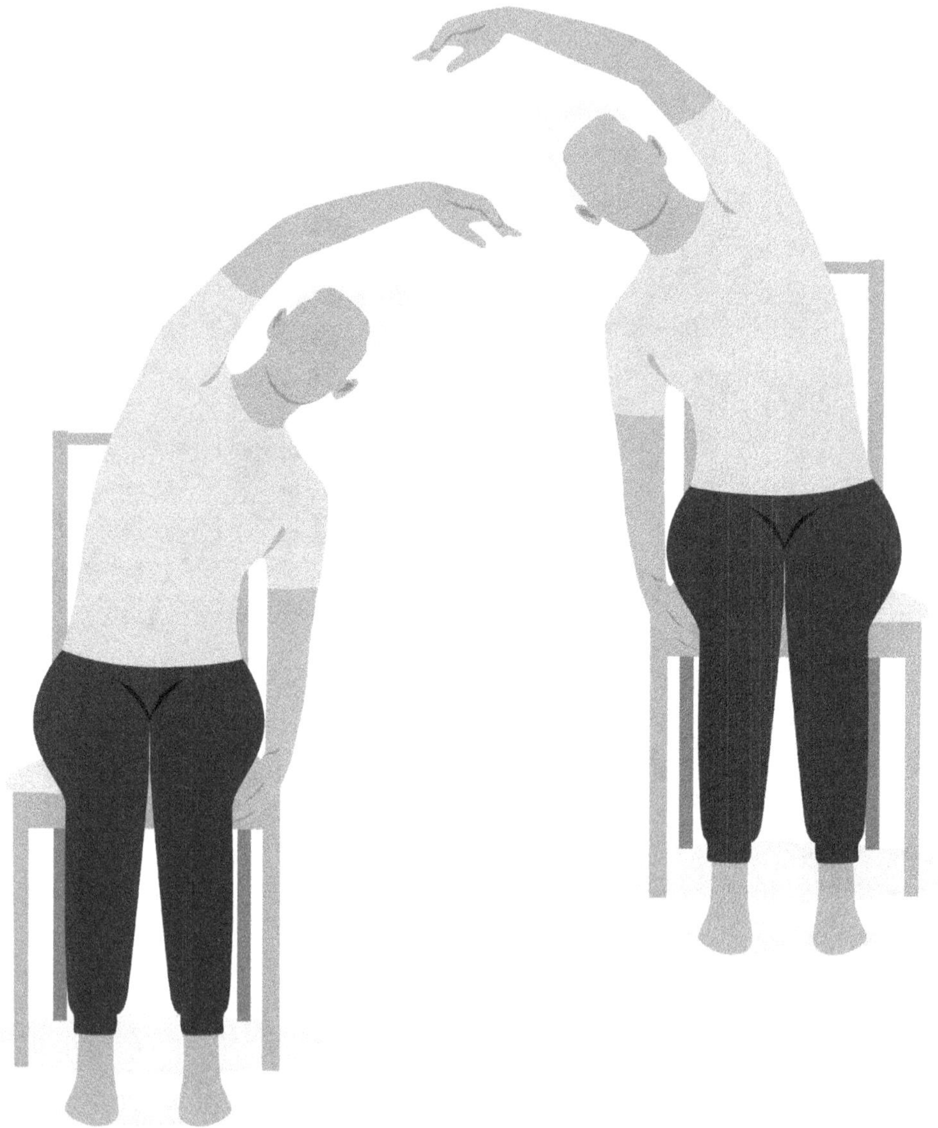

Lumbar Extensions

1. Start your practice by sitting upright in your chair and relaxing your neck and shoulders. Your feet should be flat on the floor, about hip-width apart, with your knees in line with your ankles. Your hands can be resting on your thighs.

2. Place your hands on the bottom of your back.

3. Gently lean back into your hands and slightly arch your back.

4. Hold for as long as needed.

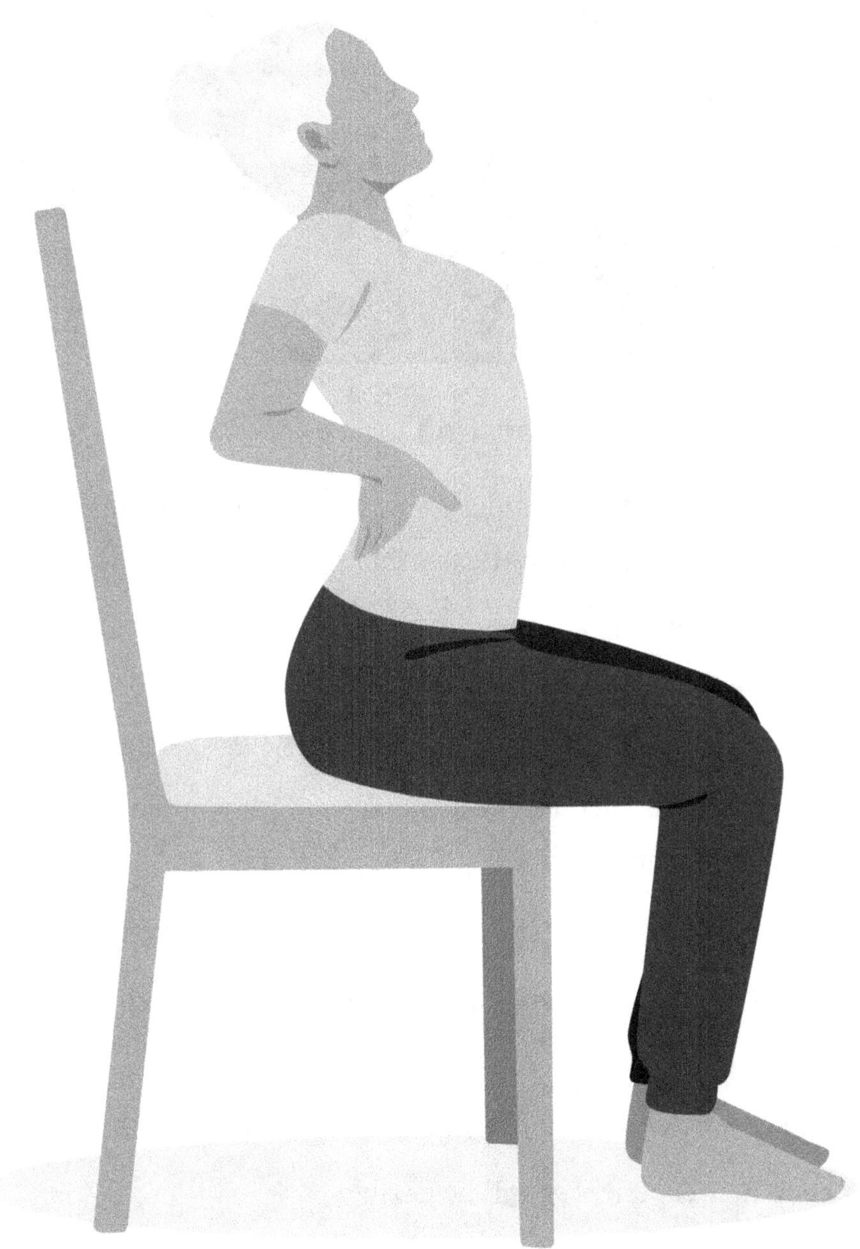

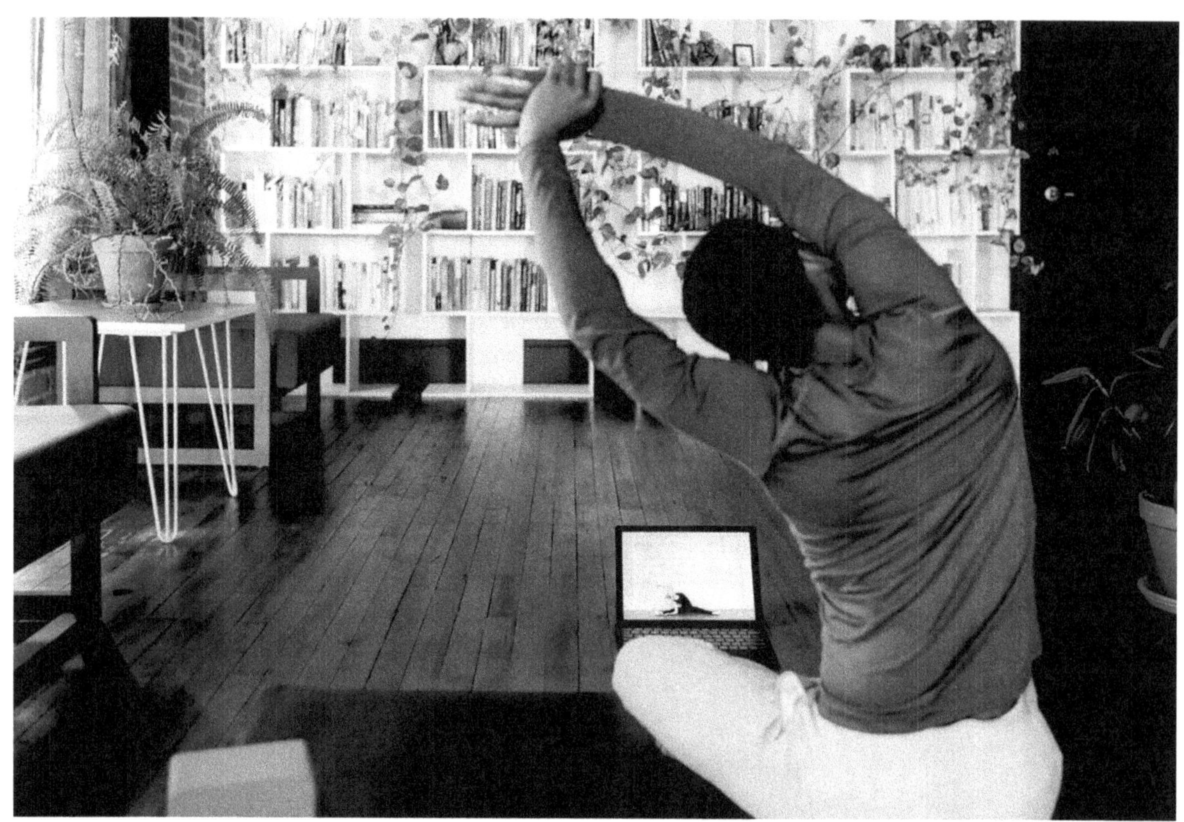

Guided Imagery and Mental Preparation

We know that yoga is as much a mental endeavor as it is physical. The main goal is to merge body and mind, creating a connection between the two and creating holistic well-being.

Yoga encourages mindfulness, and in today's fast-paced world, this is a much-needed and welcome reset. Mindfulness encourages us to be present, open, and receptive to what is happening around us. This can lead to an increased sense of peace, calm, and a positive outlook on life.

Here are some ways that you can mentally prepare yourself for your yoga session and get the most out of the mental benefits of your practice:

- Regularly practice mindfulness in your daily activities and when not practicing.

- Set intentions for your practice and know what you want to achieve so that you can guide your experience.

- Be mindful of self-care and look after your physical, mental, and emotional well-being.

- Remain open to new experiences and be flexible.

Guided Imagery

By utilizing all five of our senses along with positive self-talk and affirmations, we can use our imagination to create positive mind/body effects. This guided imagery script was adapted from Taking Charge (n.d.).

Guided Visualization Script One

1. Sit back and unwind on a chair, on the floor, or on a bed.

2. Tune in and focus on your breath. Take a few deep breaths in and out. Allow each inhalation to become deeper and each exhale to linger a little bit longer as you breathe into your abdomen.

3. With each inhale and exhale, you begin to release discomfort, tension, anxiety, and distraction. You begin to release feelings and emotions you do not need to hold onto.

4. Your breath begins to transport you to a place of peace, comfort, and beauty.

5. Continue to breathe deeply. In and out, in and out...

6. Imagine that you are being taken to a place of comfort and peace. A place that is special to you. It can be real, or it can be a place that is in your imagination. All the sounds that are outside of you are melting away into the background. They are not important.

7. Look around your special place and notice the colors, sounds, shapes, and other things that you see there.

8. Inhale and exhale... Do you smell anything? There may be a familiar fragrance that you are aware of. Notice it and name it if it is there.

9. Draw your attention to the weather. What is the temperature? Is it hot or cool? Sunny or cloudy?

10. Inhale and exhale deeply as you embrace the feelings of relaxation, peacefulness, and comfort. You have no obligations but to sink into these feelings and allow yourself to be here fully. Allow your body and mind to recharge and reset. You are safe. Draw from this deep well of relaxation and comfort.

11. Acknowledge that you can return to this place whenever you need to. All you have to do is shift your attention and your breath and imagine yourself here.

12. Inhale and exhale deeply. When you are ready, slowly bring yourself to your present moment by beginning to focus on the environment around you. As you allow your images to fade, continue to hold onto the feelings of peace, relaxation, safety, and calm that you experienced in your special place. This place is always within you, and the feelings it has brought on can be accessed by simply conjuring up its image in your mind.

Guided Visualization Script Two

This guided imagery script was adapted from Nash (2022).

1. Relax in a comfortable position on the floor, in a chair, or on a bed.

2. Encourage your body to release any tension and connection to the outside world and relax.

3. Start to pay attention to your breathing. Inhale and exhale deeply, and with each breath, notice how your body responds. How do your body and mind react to each breath? Each breath out invites your body to relax and soften itself.

4. Do you notice how effortless your breathing is? The automatic process brings life so easily. You do not even have to think about it. Give thanks for your breath, and let this feeling grow as you breathe, knowing that it is giving you life.

5. Now shift your focus to include your heartbeat. Put one hand over your heart and notice the beating; acknowledge that this too is automatic and your heart keeps you alive effortlessly. Feel gratitude for this miracle of life.

6. Continue to inhale and exhale as you focus on your breath and your heartbeat, two of our most important life-giving functions.

7. Now imagine a part of nature that you are most drawn to. Picture yourself in this part of nature. It could be the beach, the ocean, a river, or the mountains.

8. As you breathe in and out, not only visualize your favorite thing in nature but also express your gratitude for it.

9. If it is the mountains, imagine you are climbing up a peak. If it is the beach, imagine you are feeling the waves lap at your feet as they break on the shore.

10. Each breath in and out should invite your heart to expand with gratitude for the beauty of nature and the miracle of life. You should be filled with gratitude for your life, all you are, and the wonderful journey you are on.

11. When you are ready, take a deep breath in and breathe out completely as you prepare to come back into the present room.

12. You will emerge relaxed, refreshed, and focused.

13. Gently open your eyes.

Visualization is an important component of any meditation practice and can be another beneficial tool to use alongside your yoga practice for your mental health.

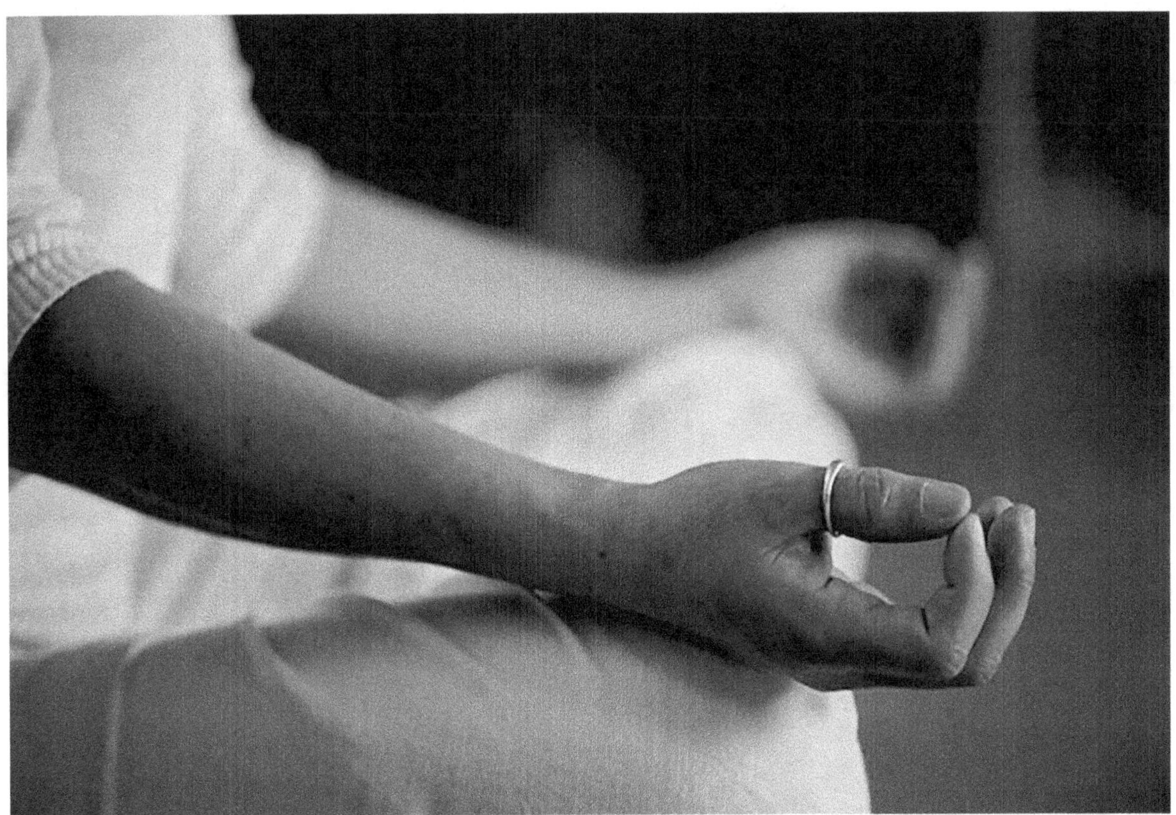

Key Takeaways

- A comprehensive warm-up routine is crucial for preparing the body and mind for yoga practice, and establishing the right foundation for a productive session.

- Yoga serves as a gateway to harmonizing the physical and mental aspects of well-being, promoting a holistic approach to health and vitality.

- Mindfulness practices within yoga advocate for being present, open, and receptive, fostering a sense of calm, peace, and optimism amid the challenges of modern-day living.

- Utilizing guided imagery and visualization techniques can enhance the mental benefits of yoga, empowering individuals to leverage their imagination for positive mind-body effects and mental wellness.

CHAPTER 4

Building Blocks of Chair Yoga

Introduction to Chair Yoga Poses

These are 10 basic yoga poses that should be mastered as a beginner, as they are found in most styles of yoga, be it Vinyasa, Hatha, or chair yoga.

These poses have been adapted for chair yoga, along with instructions on how to perform them. You can work your way through these poses intentionally as you slowly add them to your practice the more proficient you become. The same concept applies to the time frame of each exercise—this is unique and needs to be based on your own capabilities and fitness levels.

Chair Mountain Pose

Difficulty Level: Beginner

Benefits:

- Improves posture by aligning the spine, enhancing comfort during daily activities.

- Enhances body awareness, helping you maintain better alignment and reduce strain during everyday movements.

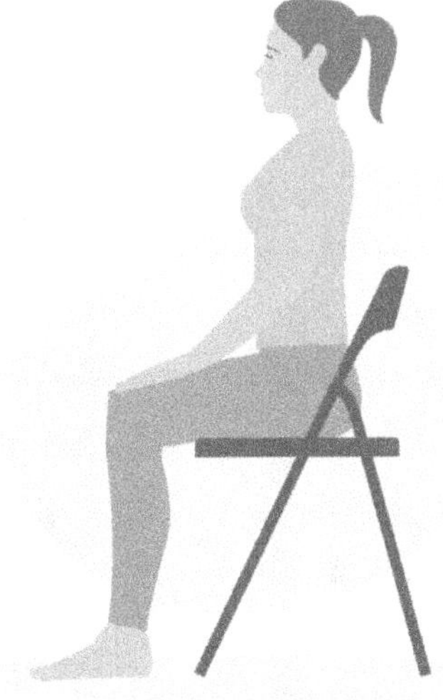

1. Start your practice by sitting upright in your chair and relaxing your neck and shoulders. Your feet should be flat on the floor, about hip-width apart, with your knees in line with your ankles. Your hands can be resting on your thighs.

2. Elongate your spine by raising your chest and dropping your shoulders.

3. Take a deep breath in through your nose and close your eyes; your air should expand into your belly.

4. Breathe out slowly through your mouth while focusing on releasing tension.

5. Keep your breath even as you ground yourself by imagining that roots are growing into the ground from your feet.

6. Stay here for as long as desired before gently opening your eyes.

Chair Downward-Facing Dog

Difficulty Level: Beginner

Benefits:

- Stretches the back and legs, reducing tension and discomfort from prolonged sitting or standing.

- Improves overall flexibility, making movements like bending and reaching easier.

- Enhances circulation and energy levels, promoting greater energy and refreshment throughout the day.

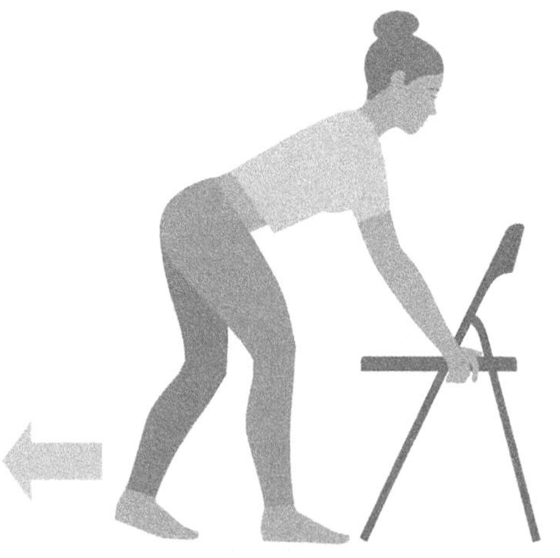
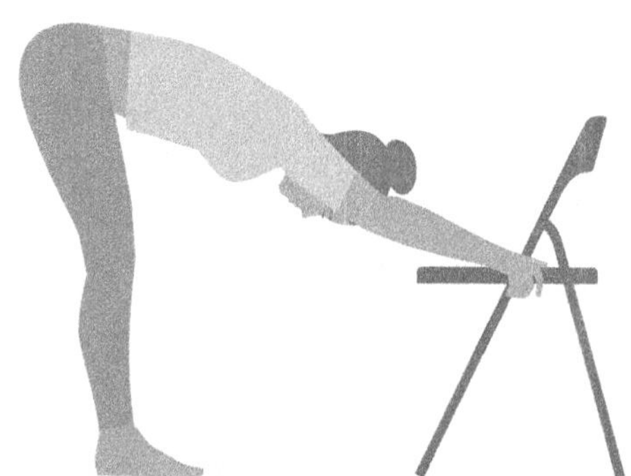

1. Start your practice by standing in front of your chair. Relax your neck and shoulders. Your feet should be hip-width apart.

2. Place your hands on the seat of your chair and carefully walk your feet backward until your body is at a 45-degree angle to the floor.

3. Breathe in and activate your midline muscles; your lower back and hips should be raised and your head and shoulders relaxed.

4. Hold this pose for as long as needed, and when you are ready to release, walk your feet back toward the chair and stand up.

Chair Upward-Facing Dog

Difficulty Level: Intermediate

Benefits:

- Opens the chest and shoulders, improving posture and making activities like sitting and standing more comfortable.

- Strengthens the upper body and core, supporting tasks that involve lifting or reaching with less effort.

- Enhances spinal flexibility, which helps in performing daily movements with greater ease and reduces back discomfort.

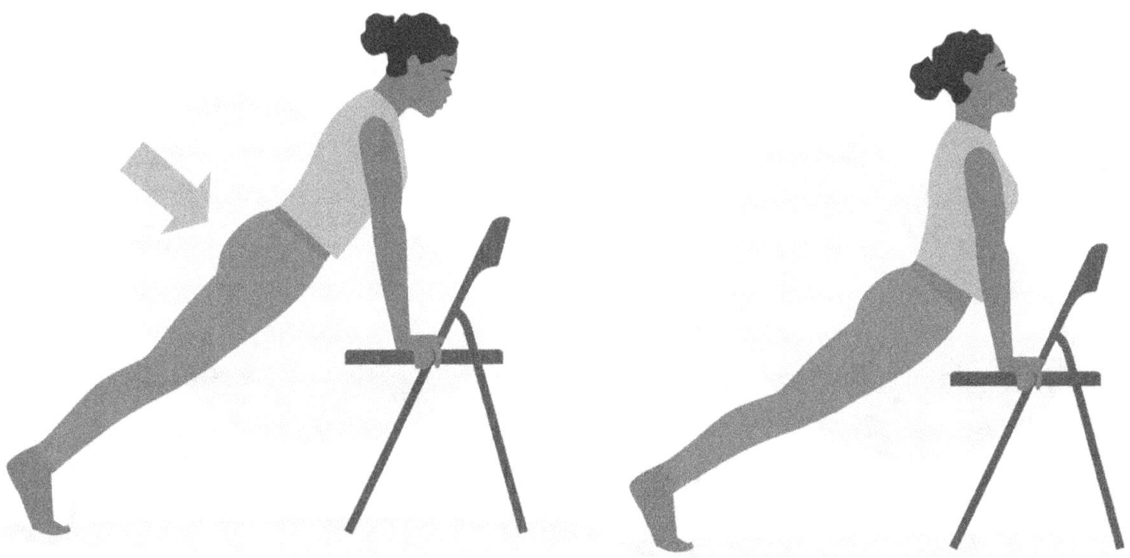

1. Start your practice by standing in front of your chair. Relax your neck and shoulders. Your feet should be hip-width apart.

2. Place your hands on the seat of your chair.

3. You want your spine to create a smooth curve. Gently push your hips forward as you arch your back and look slightly upward.

4. Carefully take a few steps backward.

5. Hold this pose for as long as needed, and when you are ready to release, walk your feet back toward the chair and stand up.

Chair Plank

Difficulty Level: Intermediate

Benefits:

- Strengthens core muscles, which improves overall stability and balance for everyday tasks like lifting or reaching.

- Enhances posture, supporting better alignment and reducing strain on the back and shoulders.

- Boosts upper body strength, making activities that involve pushing or holding objects easier and less tiring.

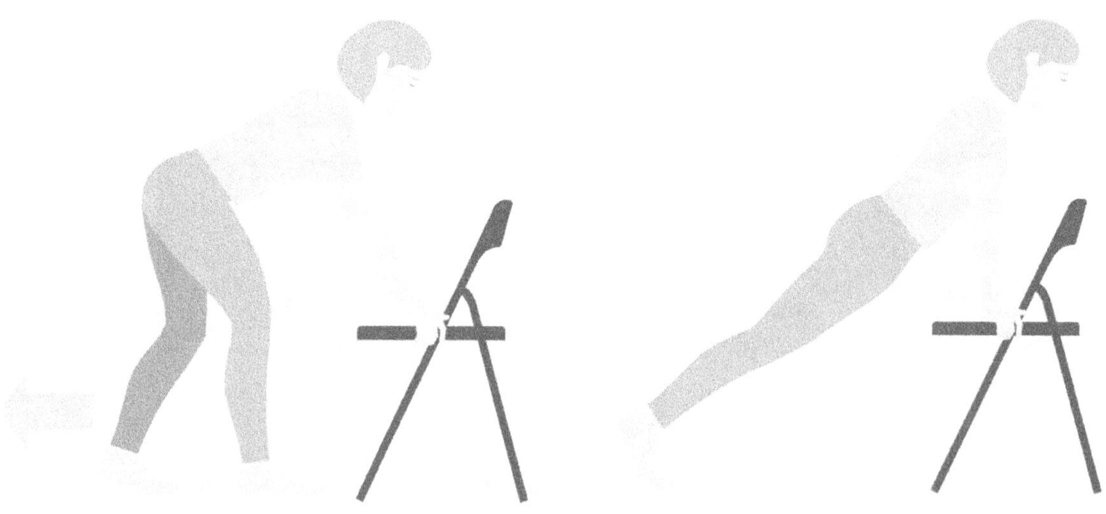

1. Start your practice by standing in front of your chair. Relax your neck and shoulders. Your feet should be hip-width apart.

2. Place your hands on the seat of your chair.

3. Walk your feet back until your body forms a straight line from the top of your head to your feet.

4. Activate your core muscles to support your body and keep your spine neutral.

5. For stability, keep your hands exactly behind your shoulders with your fingers extended wide.

6. Press into your hands as you lift your hips slightly to align your body.

7. Hold this pose for as long as needed, and when you are ready to release, walk your feet back toward the chair and stand up.

Chair Warrior One

Difficulty Level: Intermediate

Benefits:

- Strengthens legs and core, improving stability and support for activities like walking and standing.

- Enhances balance, making it easier to perform tasks that require stability, such as bending or lifting.

- Improves posture, reducing strain on the back and shoulders during daily activities.

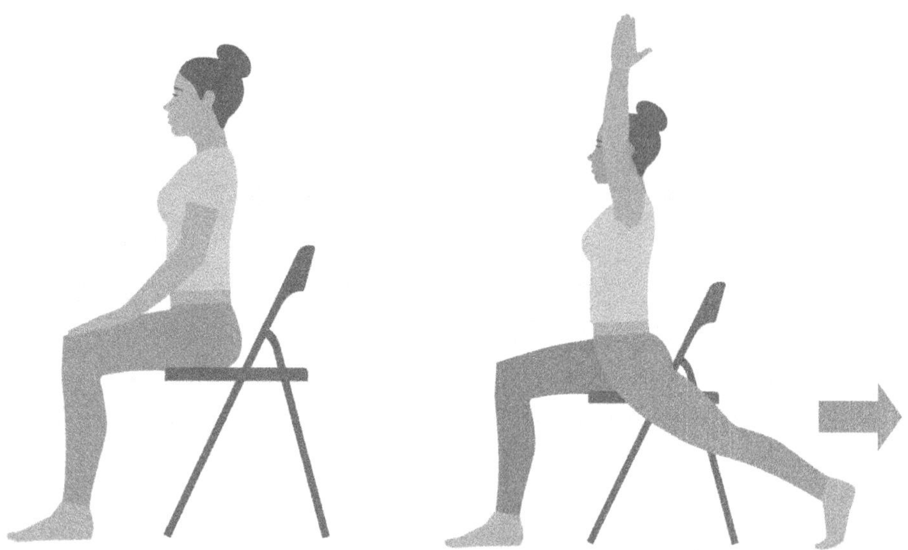

1. Start your practice by sitting upright toward the front of your chair and relaxing your neck and shoulders. Your feet should be flat on the floor, about hip-width apart, with your knees in line with your ankles. Your hands can be resting on your thighs.

2. Turn your body to the right and move your buttocks closer to the left edge of the chair. This will create support for your right thigh.

3. Stretch your left leg behind you and straighten it out as much as possible. Place the ball of your foot on the floor, keeping your heel lifted. Bend your left knee at a 90-degree angle, keeping it aligned with your ankle.

4. Raise your arms above you, reaching to the ceiling, with your palms facing each other. Alternatively, put your hands on your hips or the seat of the chair for support.

5. Keep your chest raised, and relax your shoulders. Keep your gaze forward.

6. Hold this pose for as long as needed, then release and swap sides.

Chair Warrior Two

Difficulty Level: Intermediate

Benefits:

- Strengthens legs and core, providing better stability and support for activities like walking or standing.

- Improves balance, making it easier to perform tasks that require stability, such as reaching or lifting.

- Enhances posture, reducing strain on the back and shoulders during everyday activities.

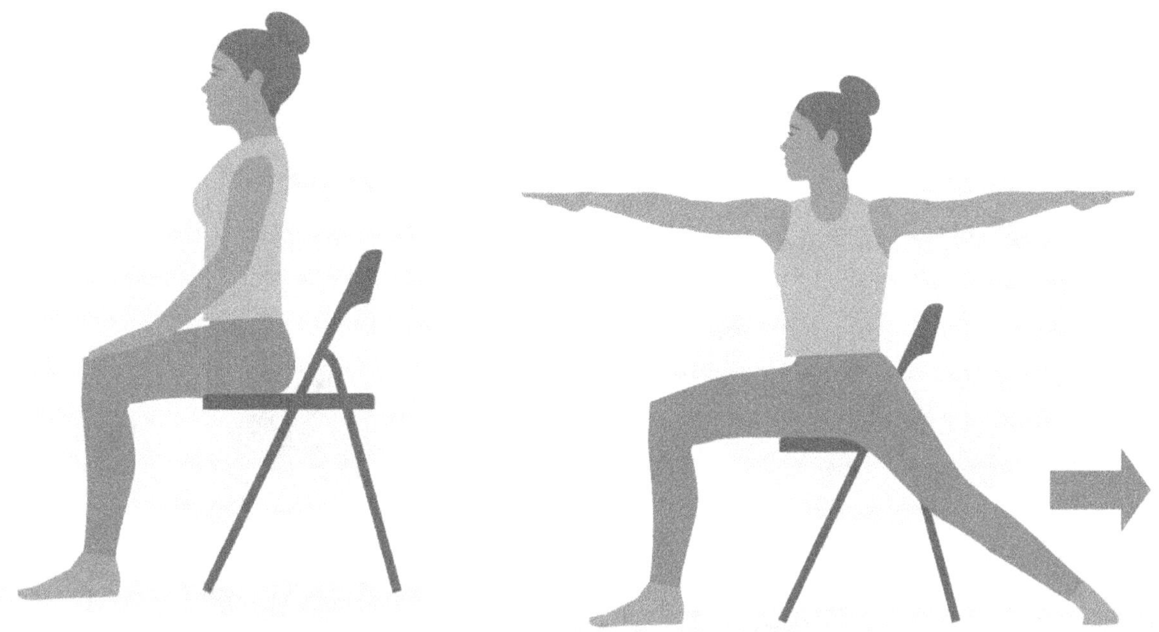

1. Start your practice by sitting upright toward the front of your chair and relaxing your neck and shoulders. Your feet should be flat on the floor, about hip-width apart, with your knees in line with your ankles. Your hands can be resting on your thighs.

2. Turn your body to the right and move your buttocks closer to the left edge of the chair. This will create support for your right thigh.

3. Stretch your left leg behind you and straighten it out as much as possible. Place the ball of your foot on the floor, keeping your heel lifted. Bend your left knee at a 90-degree angle, keeping it aligned with your ankle.

4. Raise your arms out to the sides at shoulder height, palms facing down, in a T-position.

5. Gaze over your left hand.

6. Keep your shoulders relaxed and your spine elongated.

7. Hold this pose for as long as needed, then release and swap sides.

Seated Twist

Difficulty Level: Beginner

Benefits:

- Improves spinal flexibility, making daily tasks like twisting and reaching more comfortable.

- Relieves back discomfort, reducing strain during activities such as sitting or standing for long periods.

- Enhances digestion, which can lead to improved comfort and energy throughout the day.

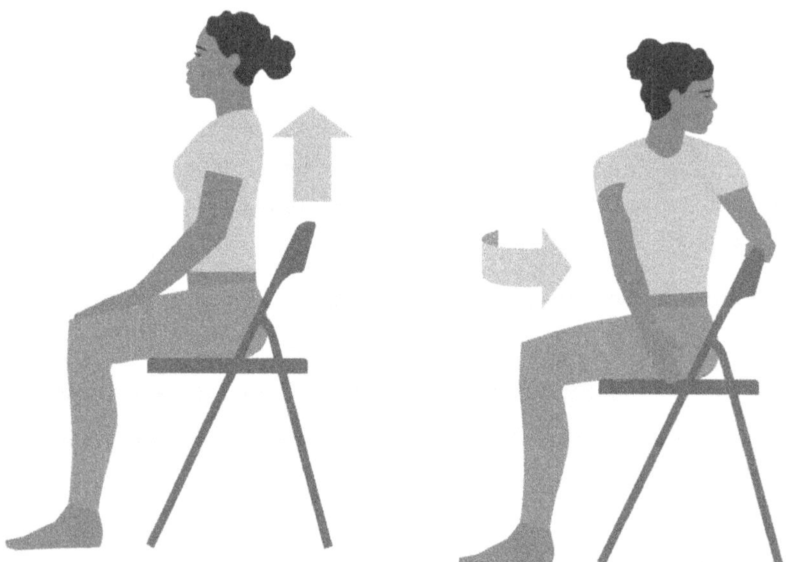

1. Start your practice by sitting upright in your chair and relaxing your neck and shoulders. Your feet should be flat on the floor, about hip-width apart, with your knees in line with your ankles. Your hands can be resting on your thighs.

2. Breathe in as you lengthen your spine, and as you breathe out, twist to the right.

3. Put your right hand on the chair's back and your left hand on the outside of your right thigh.

4. Keep your spine long and twist from your torso, not just from your shoulders.

5. Look over your right shoulder for a deeper twist.

6. Hold the twist for as long as needed.

7. Inhale to release the twist back to the center.

8. Repeat the twist on the other side by twisting to the left.

Cat Pose

Difficulty Level: Beginner

Benefits:

- Relieves back tension, reducing discomfort from prolonged sitting and making everyday activities more comfortable.

- Improves flexibility, enhancing spinal mobility to help with bending and reaching.

- Enhances core strength, boosting balance and stability, supporting better posture, and making movement tasks easier.

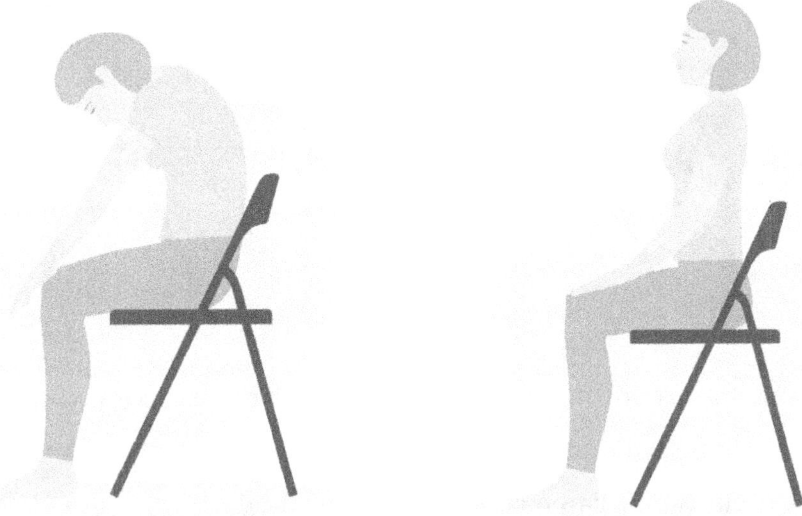

1. Start your practice by sitting upright in your chair and relaxing your neck and shoulders. Your feet should be flat on the floor, about hip-width apart, with your knees in line with your ankles. Your hands can be resting on your thighs.

2. Breathe in, round your spine, and lower your chin to your chest.

3. Breathe in and out deeply as you hold for as long as needed.

4. When you are ready to release, breathe out and slowly roll your head up to a neutral position.

Cow Pose

Difficulty Level: Beginner

Benefits:

- Improves Posture: Enhances spinal alignment for more comfortable sitting and standing.

- Reduces Back Pain: Alleviates discomfort from prolonged sitting or standing.

- Increases Flexibility: Aids in bending and reaching, making daily tasks easier.

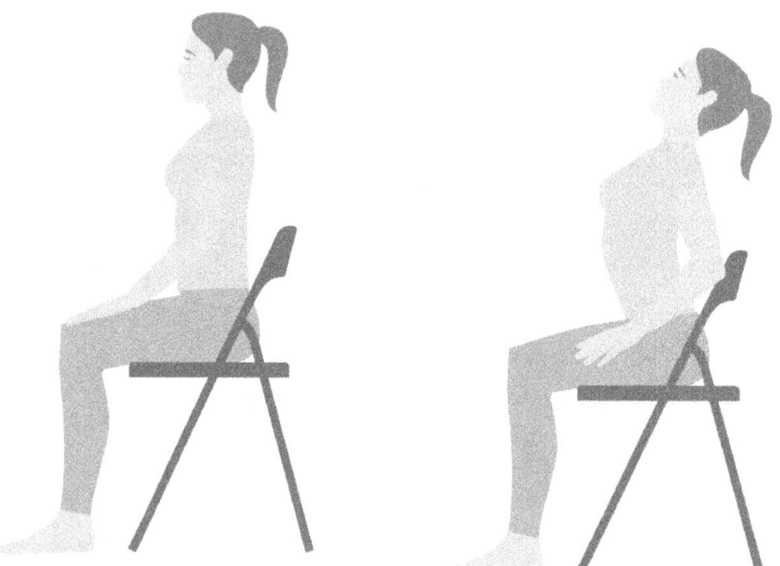

1. Start your practice by sitting upright in your chair and relaxing your neck and shoulders. Your feet should be flat on the floor, about hip-width apart, with your knees in line with your ankles. Your hands can be resting on your thighs.

2. Breathe in and arch your back while looking up at the ceiling.

3. Breathe in and out deeply as you hold for as long as needed.

4. When you are ready to release, breathe out and slowly roll your head up to a neutral position.

Happy Baby Pose

Difficulty Level: Beginner

Benefits:

- Stretches the back and hips, reducing tension and discomfort from sitting or standing for long periods.

- Relieves lower back pain, making daily activities like sitting or bending more comfortable.

- Decreases tension and encourages relaxation, making you feel more at ease and focused all day.

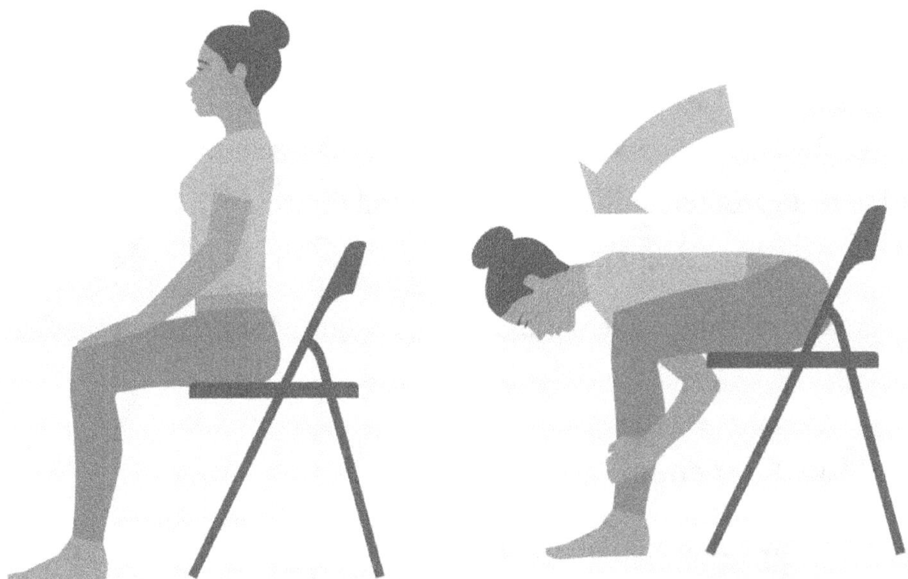

1. Start your practice by sitting upright toward the front of your chair. Relax your neck and shoulders. Your feet should be flat on the floor, a little further than hip-width apart, with your knees in line with your ankles. Your hands can be resting on your thighs.

2. Breathe in and fold forward from your waist, bringing your naval between your thighs. You may need to widen your legs to make more space for your upper body.

3. As you breathe in, reach down and take hold of your shins, ankles, or feet.

4. Carefully pull your torso down as you lower your body toward the floor.

5. Breathe in and out in this position for as long as needed.

6. When you are ready, you can release the pose by letting go of your legs and lifting your upper body back to its neutral seated position.

The Role of Alignment and Posture

When we speak of alignment, we refer to how we hold our bodies in each yoga position. Each pose has a specific way that it should be performed, and by adhering to the correct form, we can ensure that we do not get injured. We risk straining our joints or muscles if we perform these movements with incorrect alignment.

We also want to ensure that we get the maximum benefit out of our practice, which means performing the poses correctly so we are working the correct muscles.

The way we hold our bodies when we sit, stand, or lie down is known as our posture. Improper posture can lead to fatigue, muscle imbalances, pain, and discomfort. How often have you woken up with neck or back pain after sleeping in a strange position?

Correct posture when performing yoga asanas ensures that you maintain balance and stability during your practice.

Movement and Flow Sequences

You have control over how you would like to structure your yoga flow. Long or short, upper body focused or lower body focused, you can piece together a flow that suits you using the various poses in this book.

There are no rules when it comes to your practice, but there are some guidelines that you can follow to create your first flow.

- Structure your flow around a warm-up and cool-down sequence.

- Select a peak pose. This pose will be worked up to through all the poses that are performed before it, and the rest of the poses will wind down from it.

- Maintain balance by performing the same pose on each side for the same duration.

Putting Together Movements

The Chair Cat-Cow sequence consists of two complementary movements: the Cat pose and the Cow pose. This dynamic duo is perfect for introducing the concept of flow in chair yoga because it emphasizes fluid motion and coordinated breathing.

Chair Cat-Cow

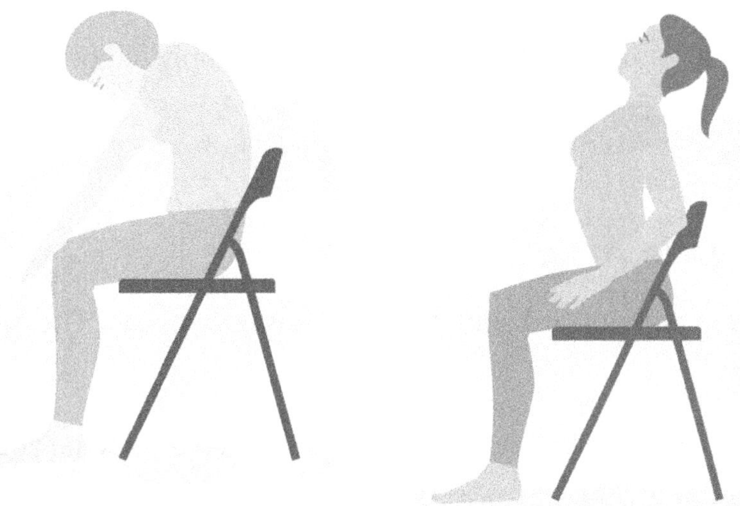

1. Start your practice by sitting upright in your chair and relaxing your neck and shoulders. Your feet should be flat on the floor, about hip-width apart, with your knees in line with your ankles. Your hands can be resting on your thighs.

2. Breathe in, round your spine, and lower your chin to your chest.

3. Breathe in and out deeply as you hold for as long as needed.

4. Reverse the movement by breathing in and arching your back while looking up at the ceiling.

5. Breathe in and out deeply as you hold for as long as needed.

6. Alternate between cat and cow for as many repetitions as needed.

Here is a simple flow that you can use for inspiration. You will need two blocks to assist you with some of the poses.

Midday Yoga Flow

1. Start your practice by sitting upright in your chair and relaxing your neck and shoulders. Your feet should be flat on the floor, about hip-width apart, with your knees in line with your ankles. Your hands can be resting on your thighs.

2. Gently bring your right ear to your right shoulder, and rotate your head in a clockwise direction.

3. Rotate for as many repetitions as required.

4. Gently bring your right ear to your right shoulder.

5. Place your right hand gently on your left ear to apply slight pressure and deepen the stretch.

6. Hold for 30 seconds.

7. Relax and swap sides.

8. Gently tuck your chin toward your chest and lower you head. The movement comes from the neck.

9. If you would like to increase the stretch, you can do so by placing your hands behind your head and gently applying pressure.

10. Hold the stretch for 30 seconds.

11. Relax and switch directions.

12. Shrug your shoulders up toward your ears.

13. Rotate them forward, down, and back around in a circular motion.

14. Repeat for 10-15 repetitions.

15. Relax and repeat in the other direction.

16. Lift your left leg, keeping your knee bent.

17. Hold for one breath and gently lower it back to the ground.

18. Repeat for 10 repetitions.

19. Swap sides and repeat.

20. Return to your seated neutral position.

21. Cross your right ankle over your left knee and keep it flexed to protect your knee.

22. Keep your right knee pointing out to the side and carefully apply pressure on your right inner thigh to deepen the stretch.

23. Stay in this position for a few breaths in and out to feel the stretch in the outer hip and glutes of the right leg.

24. To deepen the stretch, you can fold forward at your hips, maintaining a flat back and keeping your chest lifted.

25. Hold this position for a few breaths, then slowly come back to an upright position.

26. Repeat the same steps with the left ankle over the right knee to stretch the other side.

27. Open your left leg to the side, keeping your knee stacked over your ankle. Extend your right leg out to the right side.

28. Raise your arms out to either side of you, holding them at shoulder height.

29. Breathe in and out deeply before leaning your upper body to the left. Place your left hand on the chair seat or your leg.

30. Reach your right arm over your head toward the left.

31. Hold this position for two to three breaths.

32. Relax and swap sides.

33. Return to your seated neutral position.

34. Shift your body toward the front of your chair and move your feet so that they are slightly wider than hip-width apart. Turn your feet out slightly.

35. Gently fold forward from your hips and bring your palms together into a prayer pose.

36. Press your elbows into your inner legs to increase the stretch. Let your legs press back into your arms and create slight resistance. Hold for 30 seconds.

37. Lower your right hand to your right foot and rotate your chest to the left as you raise your left arm to the sky. Hold this position for three to five breaths.

38. Return to the prayer position.

39. Swap sides and repeat.

40. Alternate between left and right for 10 repetitions.

41. Return to your neutral position.

42. Keep your knees apart, but bring your feet in closer so that they are almost touching.

43. Carefully lean forward and place your hands on the floor, block, or bolster. Your knees should be close to the backs of your upper arms or touching them if possible.

44. Press your hands firmly against your block or floor and carefully raise your feet off the ground. Keep your hips on the chair.

45. Remain here for 30 seconds.

46. Breathe in as you lengthen your spine, and as you breathe out, twist to the right.

47. Put your right hand on the chair's back and your left hand on the outside of your right thigh.

48. Keep your spine long and twist from your torso, not just from your shoulders.

49. Look over your right shoulder for a deeper twist.

50. Hold for 30 seconds.

51. Inhale to release the twist back to the center.

52. Repeat the twist on the other side by twisting to the left.

53. Return to your neutral position.

54. Extend your legs out in front of you and lean back in your chair. Place your hands on your thighs, with your hands open and your palms facing the ceiling.

55. Inhale and exhale through your nose.

56. As you breathe in and breathe out, keep count and make sure that your breaths are even in duration. Or you could choose a mantra or word that you could repeat during each breath.

57. Once you get comfortable with that breathing sequence, you can add a slight pause after each inhale and exhale.

58. Continue this breathing sequence for five minutes.

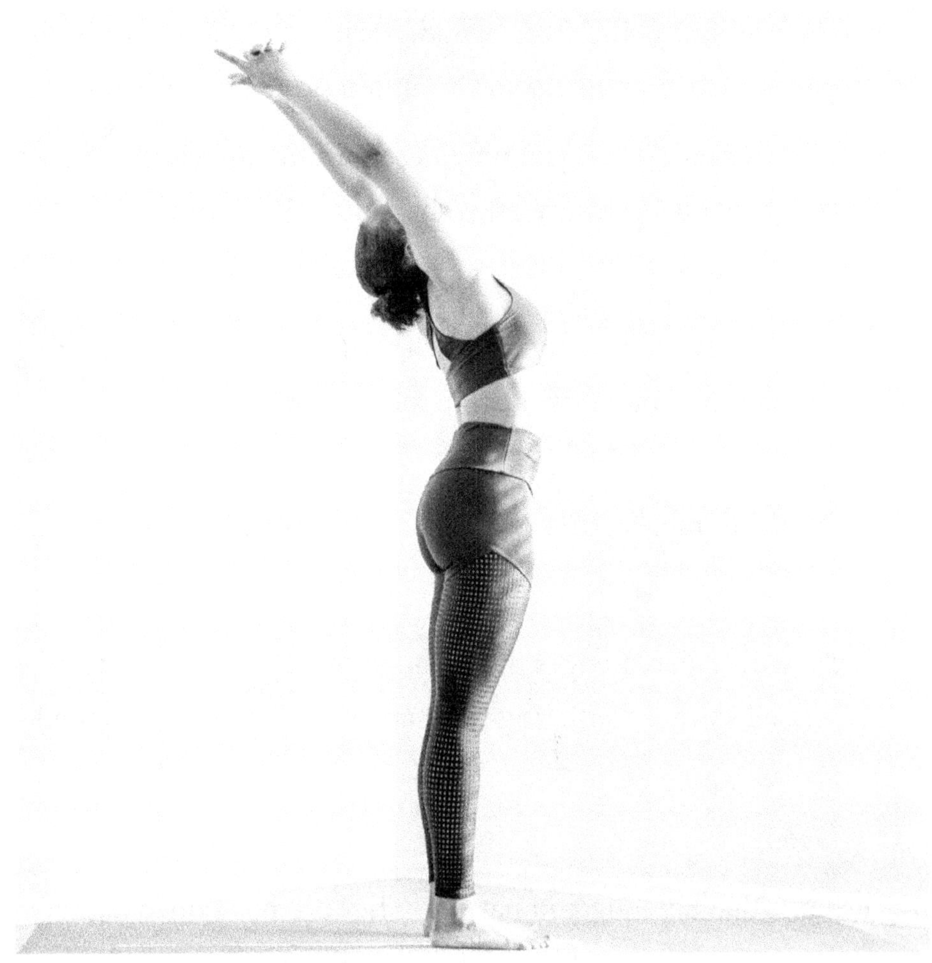

Adapting Poses for Individual Needs

In our previous flow, we made use of bolsters or blocks to modify a pose and make it easier for us to perform. Props are tools that we can use to individualize our practice and cater to our unique needs.

Yoga Mat

Your mat is the most essential yoga prop. Mats provide a stable nonslip surface and add cushioning when we come into contact with the floor.

They come in different thicknesses, and some even have guidelines on the mat to help with pose alignment and form.

Blocks

Blocks are brick-shaped and are made from wood, cork, or bamboo. They grant you greater stability, can help deepen stretches, and help you maintain proper posture and form.

They help you reduce the distance when you may need additional help reaching the floor due to flexibility issues, and they help take pressure off your joints and spine.

Straps

Straps are great for those of us who have tight muscles, particularly the hamstrings or shoulders. If a pose is outside your range of mobility, a strap allows you to perform the pose with correct alignment and form.

Straps are made from elastic durable cotton or polyester and are adjustable to fit your needs.

Wedges

Yoga wedges are blocks with tapered edges that change the angle of your feet, hands, or pelvis. These wedges are often used by those suffering from arthritis, as they offer added support to your joints.

Bolsters

Yoga bolsters are cushions that are long and narrow. They are positioned along your body where you may need extra support or accessibility. Because of their firmness, they do not lose shape when under pressure for a long period.

Blankets

Yoga blankets are used for restorative poses. They can be folded, pleated, or rolled in ways that help support you and place you in the correct alignment.

Video Recommendations

Yoga for Arthritis: Chair Yoga for Improved Mobility - Johns Hopkins Arthritis Center

https://youtu.be/yUnZzpX2KMw?si=EyJCxfIAy57Nb5VU

This video focuses on addressing morning stiffness, particularly for those with arthritis, by guiding viewers through gentle movements to warm up and lubricate the joints. It showcases sequential joint articulation exercises that can be done to improve mobility and flexibility, emphasizing the importance of regular movement for maintaining joint health.

This video can help seniors looking for chair yoga flows by providing gentle movements and stretches that can be done while seated. It demonstrates simple movements like lifting and lowering legs to improve mobility and flexibility, which is ideal for seniors. It emphasizes engaging the core muscles to protect the lower back during stretches, ensuring safe practice.

Some of the common poses performed include lifting and lowering legs, hip stretches, seated cat-cow exercises for spinal articulation, shoulder rolls, arm stretches, and side stretches. These poses focus on mobilizing and stretching different parts of the body while seated, making them accessible for a wide range of individuals.

Chair Yoga - Yoga For Seniors. Yoga With Adriene

https://youtu.be/-Ts01MC2mIo?si=NWKsi96PGxxcySBz

This video presents a chair yoga sequence led by Adriene, focusing on proper posture, breath control, and gentle movements that support mobility and flexibility. The practice emphasizes self-care and body appreciation, offering modifications for different levels of ability. The sequence includes movements targeting core strength and stability, promoting balance and flexibility in a safe and accessible way.

Some of the common poses performed in the chair yoga sequence include:

- seated mountain pose, with a focus on proper alignment and breath control

- leg extensions with toe spreading and ankle rotations for mobility and flexibility

- knee squeezes and figure 4 stretches for hip opening and flexibility

- supported warrior two pose for core strength and stability

Chair Yoga Stretch & Strength: Seated Exercises for Seniors & Beginners

https://youtu.be/gXB3NhOAalk?si=eYSiA4lDGpvHS4SR

This chair yoga workout focuses on stretches and strength exercises performed in a seated position. It underlines how crucial it is to strengthen your core, keep proper posture, and train your strength with moderate weights. The workout includes a series of yoga poses to improve flexibility, well-being, and mental health, making it suitable for individuals of all ages and fitness levels.

This video can help those looking for a chair yoga flow by:

- providing seated yoga exercises that are gentle on the joints and easy to follow, makes it suitable for older individuals with limited mobility

- incorporating strength exercises using light weights to help seniors maintain muscle mass and bone strength

- emphasizing the importance of posture and core engagement, which can improve balance and stability for seniors

- offering a variety of stretches and movements that target different muscle groups commonly affected by aging

Some of the common poses performed in the video include:

- seated forward fold

- side stretches

- figure 4 stretch

- quad stretches with leg lifts

- neck stretches

- shoulder stretches

- wrist circles and rotations

Metro Chair Yoga - "Freedom Flow"

https://youtu.be/CJej-Hz9Xf4?si=iJ4UEJfEKjcNdQKA

A sequence of beginner stretches and postures that may be performed in a chair. Emphasis is placed on breathwork, relaxation, mindfulness, and building strength and flexibility through practice. The video ends with a resting pose to promote relaxation and rejuvenation.

Based on the content, common poses performed in the video include:

- seated twists

- side body stretches

- shoulder rolls

- cat-cow movements

- warrior series poses

- hip-opening stretches

- a resting pose

In order to lower stress and enhance general wellbeing, the video focuses on breathwork and relaxation techniques. The chair yoga poses demonstrated focus on gentle movements and stretches that are safe and effective, promoting flexibility and mobility. The instructions on mindfulness and being present during the practice can help you stay focused and connected to your body. The hip-opening poses shown in the video can help you improve flexibility in the hips, which is important for mobility and balance.

Chair Yoga for Seniors, Beginners

https://youtu.be/U_jdXFfegKE?si=kY_kGV5UnP0__nic

This video is a chair yoga-inspired stretching session led by April and her mom, Aiko. They guide viewers through gentle yoga poses focusing on breathwork, flexibility, and body awareness. The workout consists of a variety of stretches and exercises that can improve flexibility, strengthen the body, and encourage relaxation. The instructors emphasize the importance of good posture and offer modifications for different levels of ability.

The video emphasizes the importance of good posture and body awareness, which are crucial for preventing injury and improving balance. The session includes breathing exercises that can help you relax and reduce stress, promoting overall well-being and mental focus. It also offers modifications for different levels of ability, making it accessible for seniors with varying mobility levels.

Some of the common poses performed include:

- head tilts with shoulder stretches

- goddess pose for thigh stretching

- modified chair pose for core engagement

- warrior one and warrior two poses for leg and hip stretches

Gentle Chair Yoga for Beginners and Seniors

https://youtu.be/1DYH5ud3zHo?si=muC3wROqZ04I19Xr

This video introduces chair yoga as a suitable practice for individuals with a limited range of motion or dealing with injuries. The instructor guides a gentle chair yoga class focusing on breath, posture, and slow movements, demonstrating various poses and stretches that can help improve strength and flexibility. By emphasizing the use of a chair with a back and providing modifications, the video ensures that the practice is safe and accessible for all levels. Additionally, the offer of a full chair yoga program provides a more in-depth exploration of chair yoga for those interested in further practice.

Common poses performed in the chair yoga class include:

- seated twists

- forward folds

- side bends

- shoulder releases

- warrior two variations

- gentle twists

- hip-opening poses

These poses are suitable for individuals of all levels and can help improve flexibility, strength, and relaxation.

Key Takeaways

- Proper alignment and posture are essential in performing yoga poses correctly to prevent injuries and maximize benefits.

- Customizing yoga flows allows you to create personalized practices catering to your preferences and needs.

- Props like blocks, straps, wedges, bolsters, and blankets aid in modifying poses and providing support for those with varying abilities.

- Yoga videos tailored for seniors and beginners focus on gentle movements, breath control, and promoting mobility and flexibility through chair yoga sequences.

- Emphasis on good posture, breathwork, and gentle movements in chair yoga practices can enhance strength, flexibility, and relaxation for individuals of all levels.

CHAPTER 5

Enhancing Flexibility, Strength & Balance

The Importance of Flexibility for Seniors

If you do not utilize your flexibility, you are more likely to see a reduction in it. This has a negative knock-on effect on other areas of your life. It's not about contorting yourself into interesting shapes with your body but maintaining healthy movement patterns.

Flexibility refers to your joints' ability to move through their full range of motion and the effectiveness of your muscles and tendons to lengthen and shorten during movement (Kinshipe Pointe, 2021).

The better your flexibility, the more effective your movement. There are many advantages of being flexible. Flexibility allows you to continue to complete your daily tasks with ease, keeping you functionally fit. It reduces your risk of getting injured and helps you maintain your balance and stability. Additionally, your posture will improve.

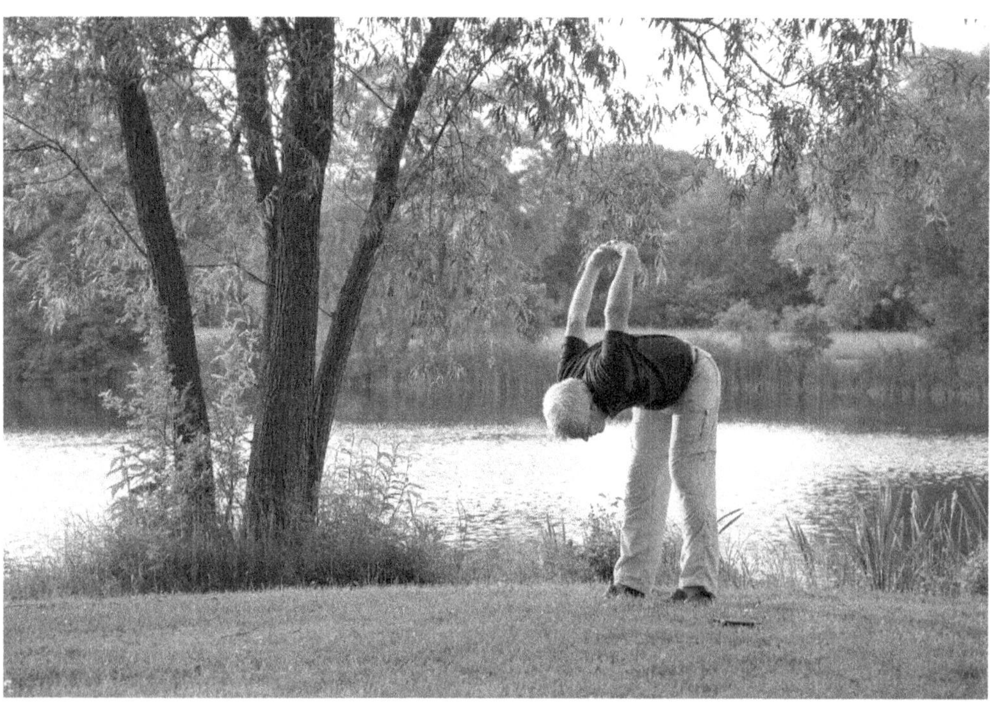

Flexibility Exercises

Remember some of these tips before getting into your stretching.

- Only stretch as far as you feel tension. You do not want to push so far that you feel pain, as this could cause injury.

- Do not bounce or jerk while stretching; rather, hold the stretch comfortably.

- Keep your joints soft and do not lock them.

- The average time to hold your stretch is 30 seconds.

- Do not hold your breath; rather, maintain a steady breathing pattern (Kinshipe Pointe, 2021).

Triceps Stretches

1. Start your practice by sitting upright toward the front of your chair and relaxing your neck and shoulders. Your feet should be flat on the floor, about hip-width apart, with your knees in line with your ankles. Your hands can be resting on your thighs.

2. Raise your right arm overhead, keeping it in line with your ear. Bend your elbow. Your palm should be flat against your upper back, between your shoulder blades, and your elbow should be pointing toward the ceiling.

3. Use your left hand to gently press on your right elbow, adding a slight stretch to your triceps.

4. Hold the stretch for 15-30 seconds, breathing deeply.

5. Repeat on the other side with your left arm.

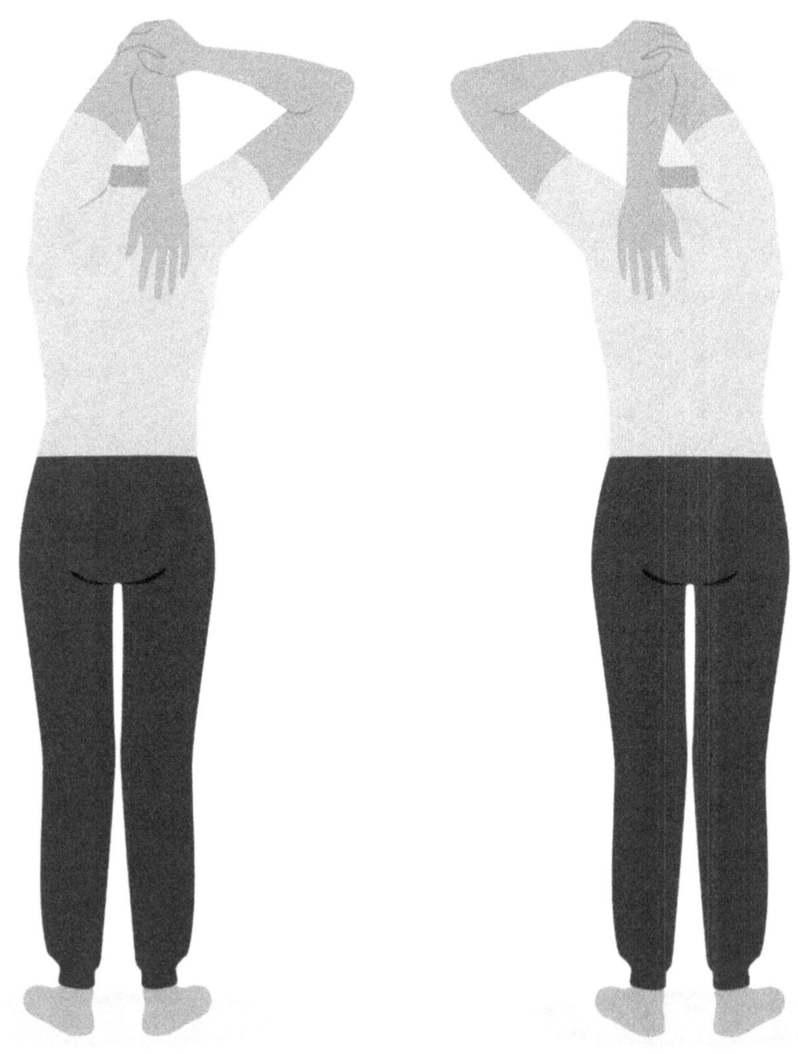

Overhead Side Stretches

1. Start your practice by sitting upright in your chair and relaxing your neck and shoulders. Your feet should be flat on the floor, about hip-width apart, with your knees in line with your ankles. Your hands can be resting on your thighs.

2. Raise your left arm overhead, keeping it in line with your ears.

3. Reach to the right, keeping your torso facing forward.

4. Hold for 30 seconds.

5. Swap arms and repeat.

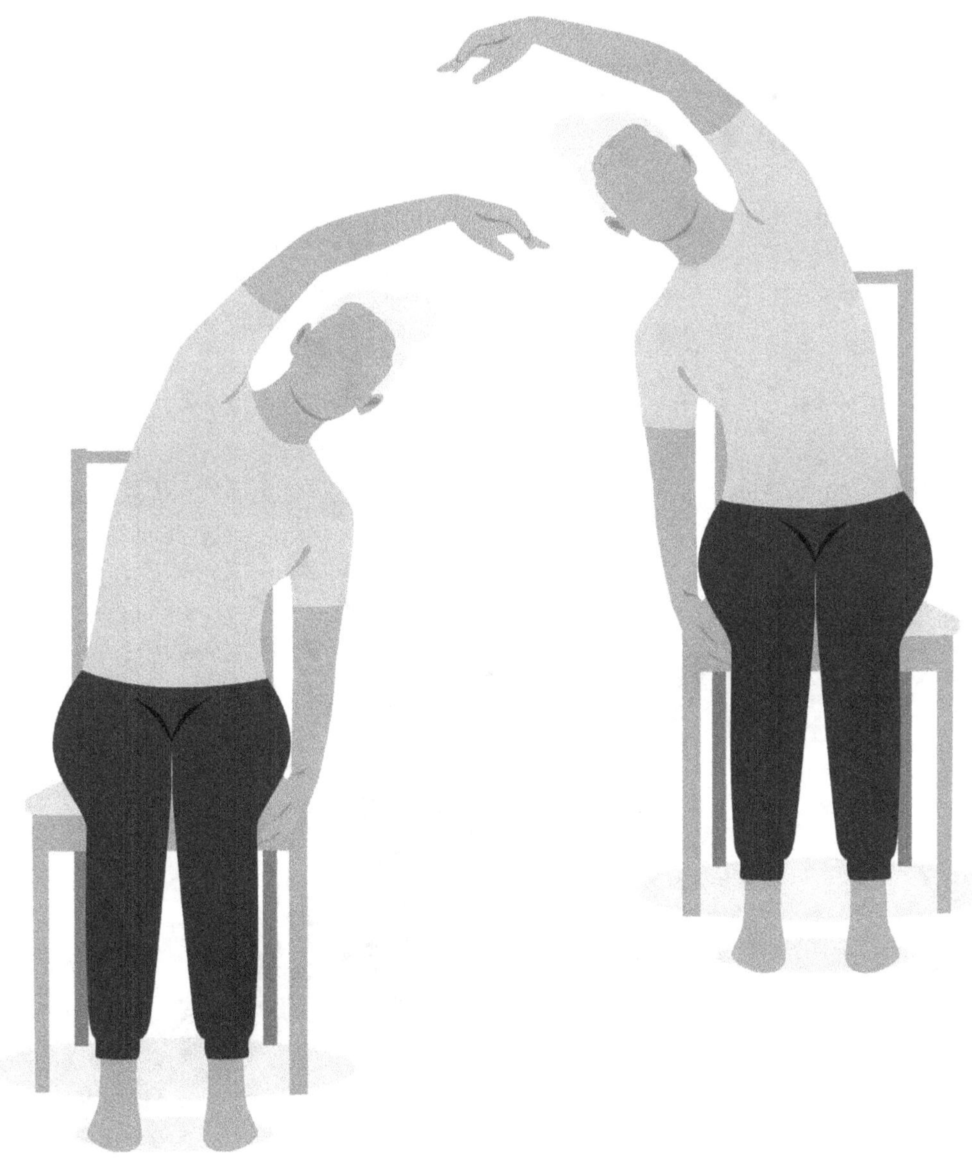

Hamstring Stretches

1. Start your practice by sitting upright toward the front of your chair and relaxing your neck and shoulders. Your feet should be flat on the floor, about hip-width apart, with your knees in line with your ankles. Your hands can be resting on your thighs.

2. Extend your left leg out in front of you, keeping your right bent at the knee.

3. Bend forward from your hips and carefully slide your hands down your left leg as you feel a stretch in your hamstring. Extend as far as you feel comfortable.

4. Hold for 30 seconds.

5. Swap sides and repeat on your right side.

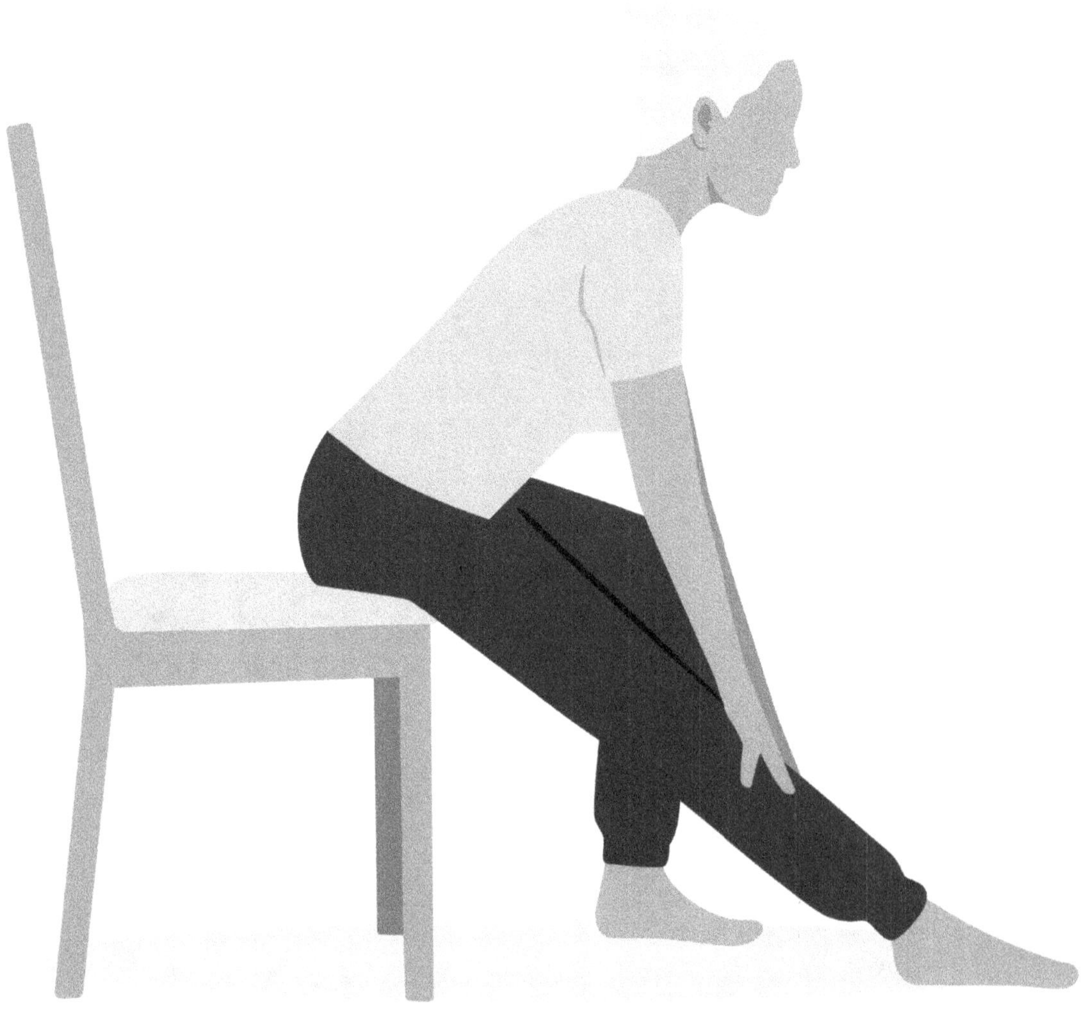

Back Extensions

1. Start your practice by sitting upright in your chair and relaxing your neck and shoulders. Your feet should be flat on the floor, about hip-width apart, with your knees in line with your ankles. Your hands can be resting on your thighs.

2. Interlace your fingers behind your neck, with your elbows out to your sides and wide.

3. Lean back on the backrest of your chair while arching your back and pushing your chest out in front of you.

4. Hold this position for 10-15 seconds.

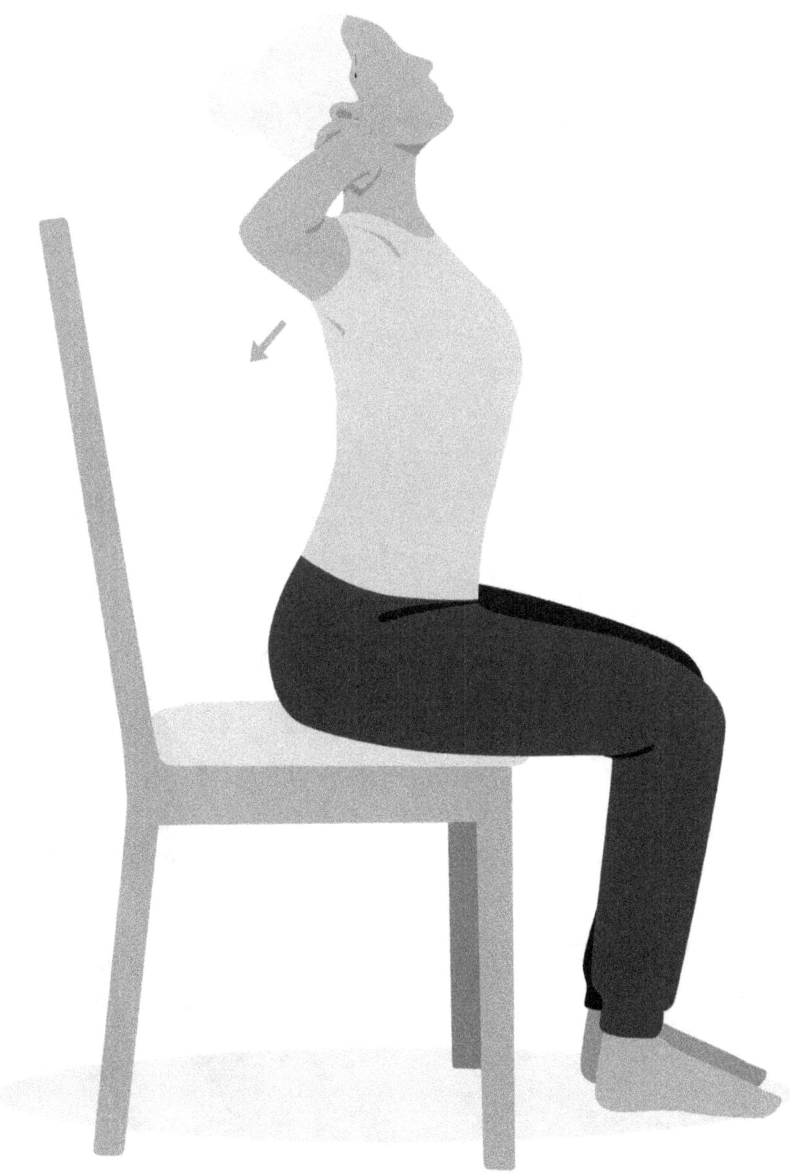

Standing Side Bends

1. Begin by standing upright behind your chair. Relax your shoulders and your neck. Keep your feet about hip-width apart.

2. Cross one of your legs behind the other, stepping back quite a bit.

3. Raise your opposite arm over your head and lean over to the side, pushing out your hip as you do so.

4. You can hold onto the back of your chair for support.

5. Hold for 15 seconds while continuing to breathe deeply.

6. Release and return to the center.

7. Repeat for as many repetitions as required.

8. Swap sides and repeat.

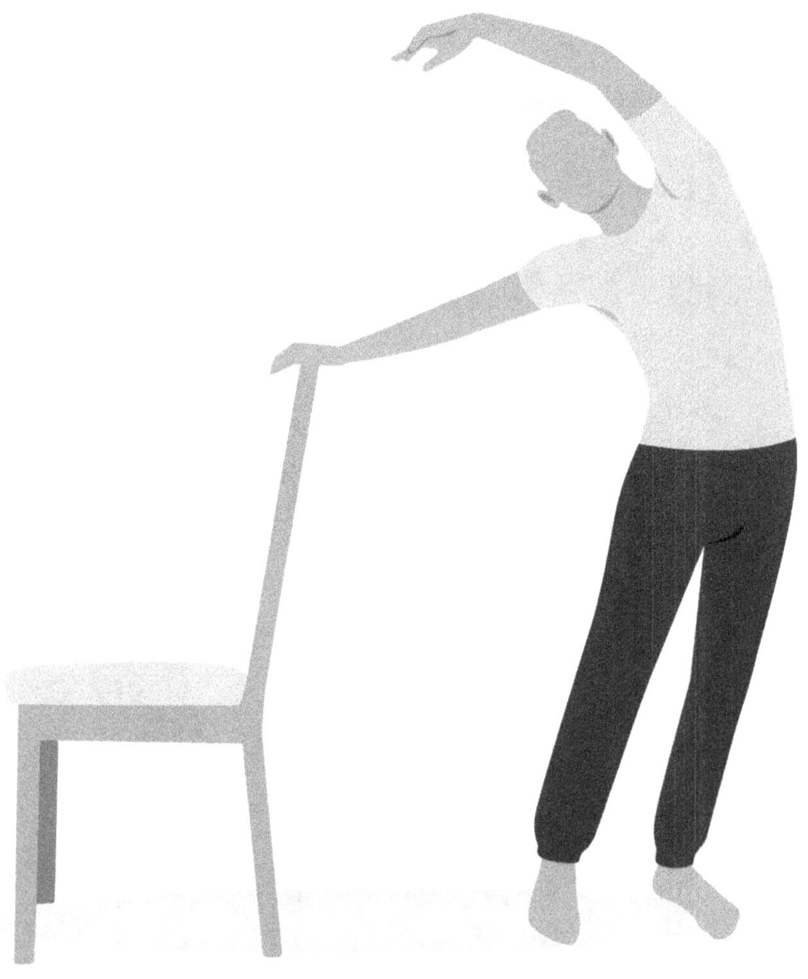

Chair Shoulder Stretches

1. Begin by standing upright behind your chair. Relax your shoulders and your neck. Keep your feet about hip-width apart.

2. Take a step back from your chair and bend forward from your hips. Rest your hands on the back of the chair; they should be almost straight, with a slight bend in the elbow.

3. Lower your chest further down to feel a stretch in your shoulders and the back of your legs.

4. Hold for as long as needed.

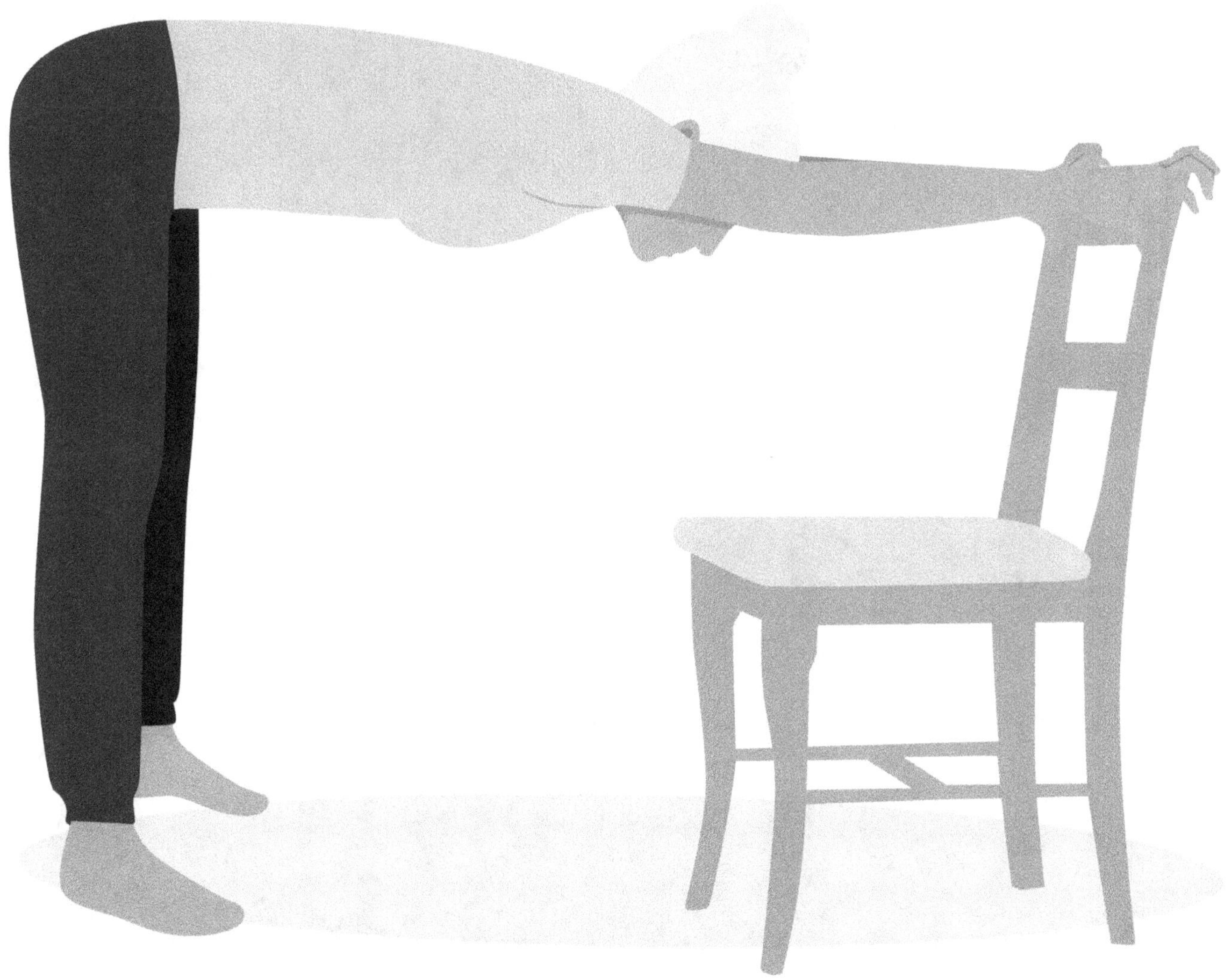

Strength-Building Exercises

As we get older, we begin to lose strength as our muscle mass decreases. It is very important that we work to maintain and continue to build muscle. We can do this by using chair yoga to build strength.

According to Davis (2021), we lose muscle mass at a rate of 3-8 percent per decade after age 30. After 60 years of age, this rate increases. This is known as sarcopenia, and its onset can increase our risk of falls and injury.

Apart from maintaining muscle mass and reducing our risk of sarcopenia, strength training has a range of other benefits, such as:

- promoting better balance

- improving body composition

- increasing bone density

- improving quality of life

Upper Body Strength: Arm and Shoulder Exercises

Shoulder Press-Ups

1. Start your practice by sitting upright in your chair and relaxing your neck and shoulders. Your feet should be flat on the floor, about hip-width apart, with your knees in line with your ankles. Your hands can be resting on your thighs.

2. Keeping your elbows bent, raise your arms to the side of you in line with your shoulders, with your palms facing forward. You will create a goalpost with your arms.

3. Lift your hands above your head, focusing on keeping your shoulder blades active.

4. Lower them back down to the starting position.

5. Repeat for as many repetitions as required.

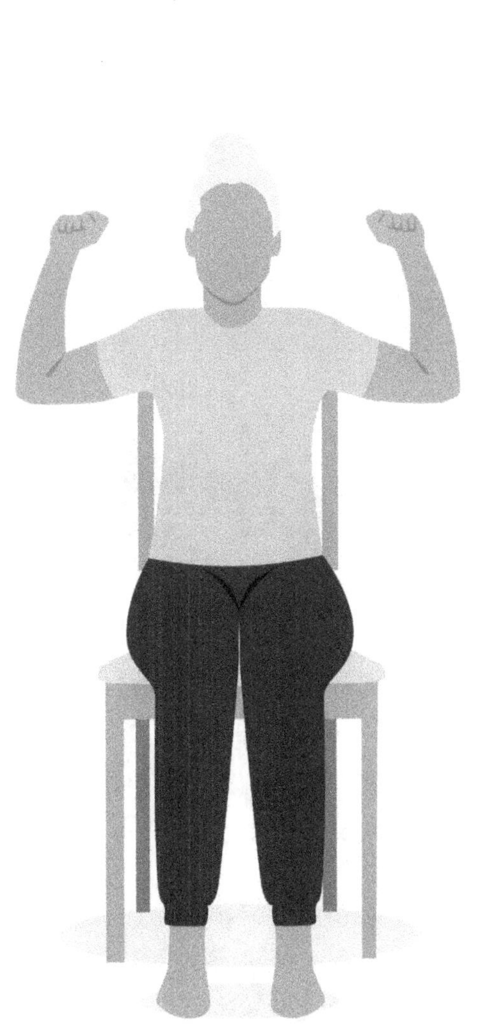
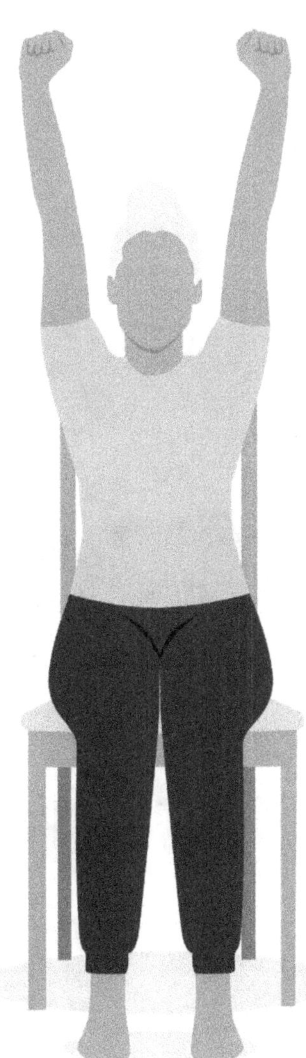

Shoulder Flexions

1. Start your practice by sitting upright in your chair and relaxing your neck and shoulders. Your feet should be flat on the floor, about hip-width apart, with your knees in line with your ankles. Your hands can be resting on your thighs.

2. Place your arms at your side, with your thumbs facing forward.

3. Raise your arms as high as they can go, keeping them straight.

4. Slowly bring them back down to the starting position.

5. Repeat for as many repetitions as required.

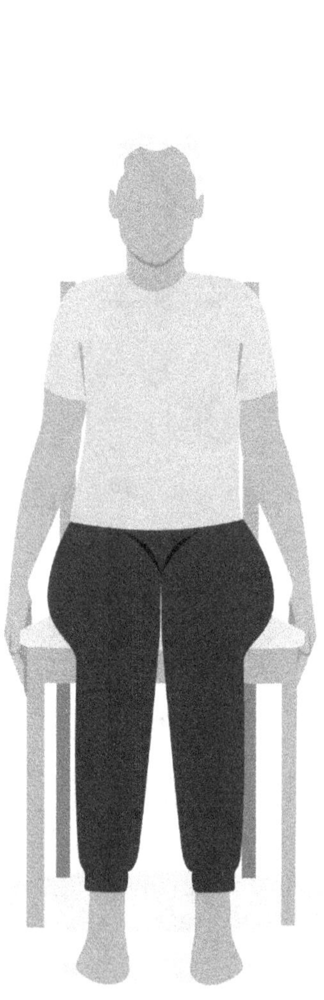
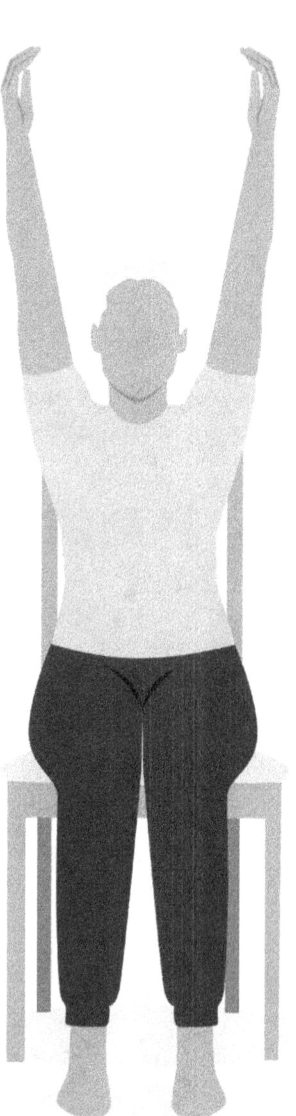

Seated Rows

1. Start your practice by sitting upright toward the front of your chair and relaxing your neck and shoulders. Your feet should be flat on the floor, about hip-width apart, with your knees in line with your ankles. Your hands can be resting on your thighs.

2. Raise your arms out in front of you at shoulder height.

3. Squeeze your shoulder blades together at the end of the action while slowly bringing your elbows back behind you.

4. Keep your chest up throughout this exercise.

5. Repeat for as many repetitions as required.

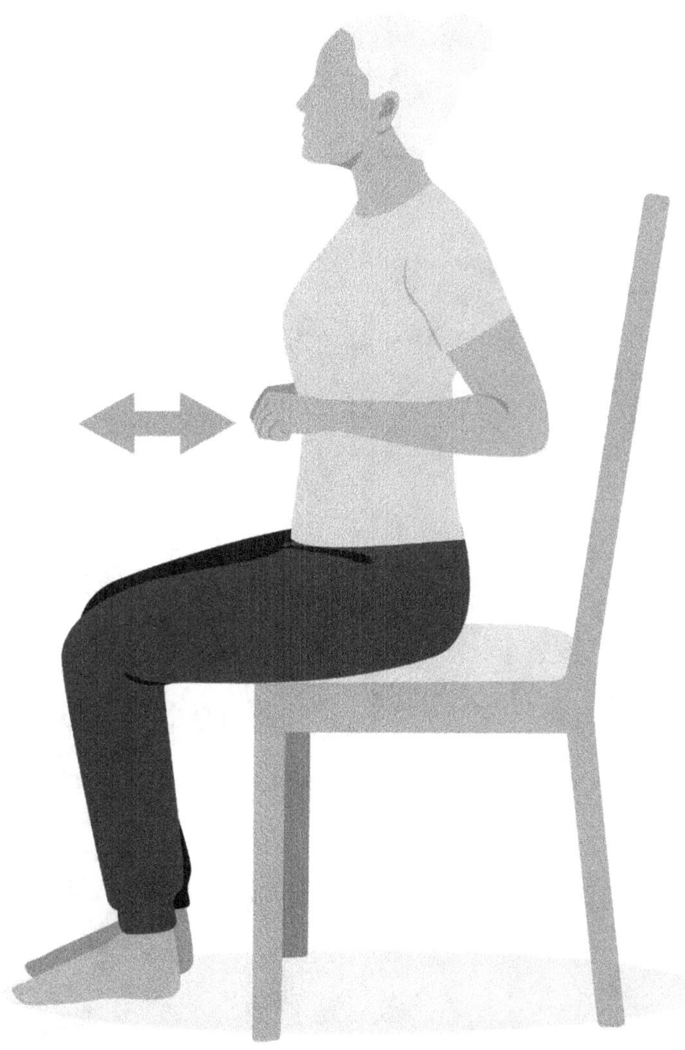

Core Strength: Abdominal and Back Exercises

Oblique Twists

1. Start your practice by sitting upright in your chair and relaxing your neck and shoulders. Your feet should be flat on the floor, about hip-width apart, with your knees in line with your ankles. Your hands can be resting on your thighs.

2. Bring your hands up to your shoulders and place your fingertips on your shoulders, keeping your elbows out to the side.

3. Gently rotate your upper body to the left, as far as you feel comfortable.

4. Rotate to your right.

5. Continue twisting from left to right for as many repetitions as required.

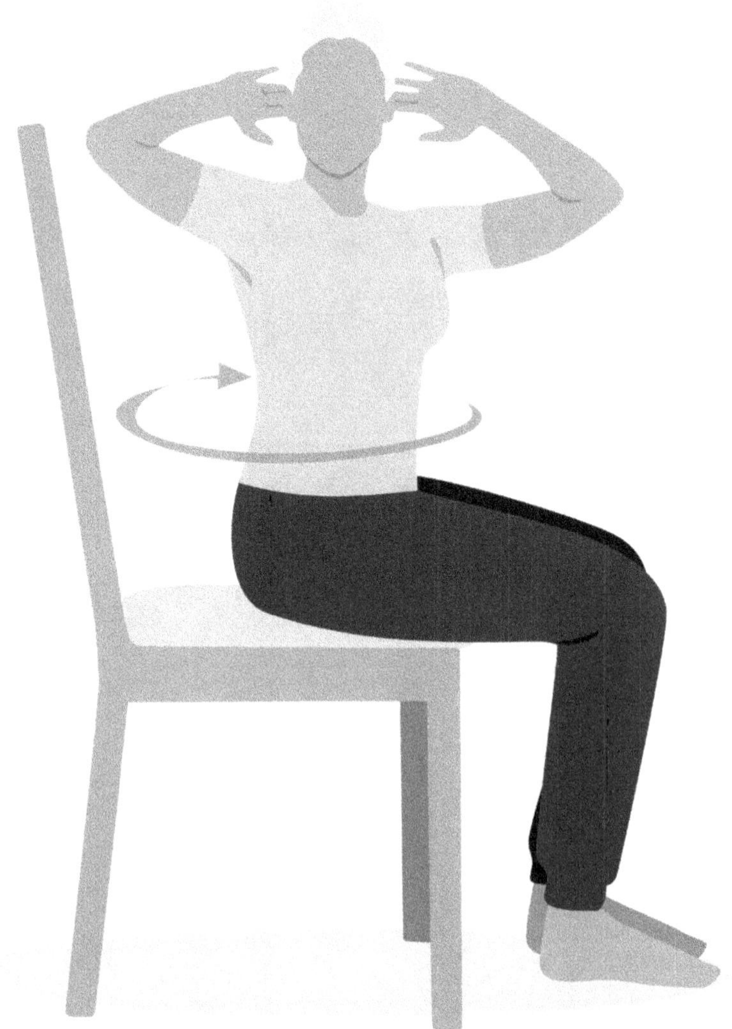

Alternate Bicycle Crunches

1. Start your practice by sitting upright in your chair and relaxing your neck and shoulders. Your feet should be flat on the floor, about hip-width apart, with your knees in line with your ankles. Your hands can be resting on your thighs.

2. Place both your hands behind your head, with your elbows facing out to the side.

3. Gently rotate your upper body and bring your left elbow gently across your body to the right.

4. Lift your right leg up simultaneously, keeping the knee bent.

5. Release and return to the center.

6. Gently rotate your upper body and bring your right elbow gently across your body to the left.

7. Lift your left leg up simultaneously, keeping the knee bent.

8. Repeat for as many repetitions as required.

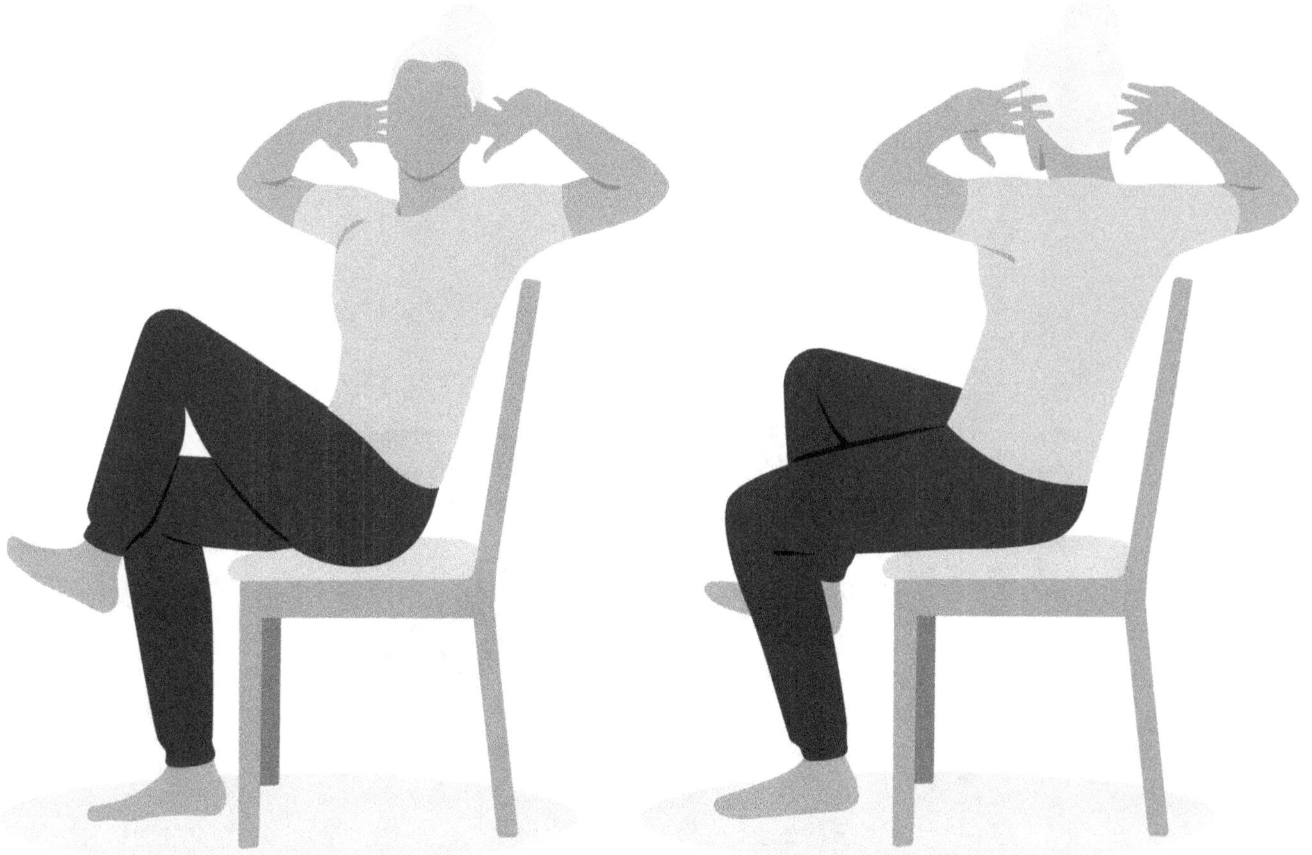

Butterfly Kicks

1. Start your practice by sitting upright in your chair and relaxing your neck and shoulders. Your feet should be flat on the floor, about hip-width apart, with your knees in line with your ankles. Your hands can be resting on your thighs.

2. Keeping both legs straight, raise them in front of you as high as you feel comfortable.

3. Raise your arms straight in front of you at shoulder height.

4. Gently flutter kick your legs, keeping them straight as you do so.

5. If you feel comfortable, you can do the same with your arms.

6. Continue for as long as needed.

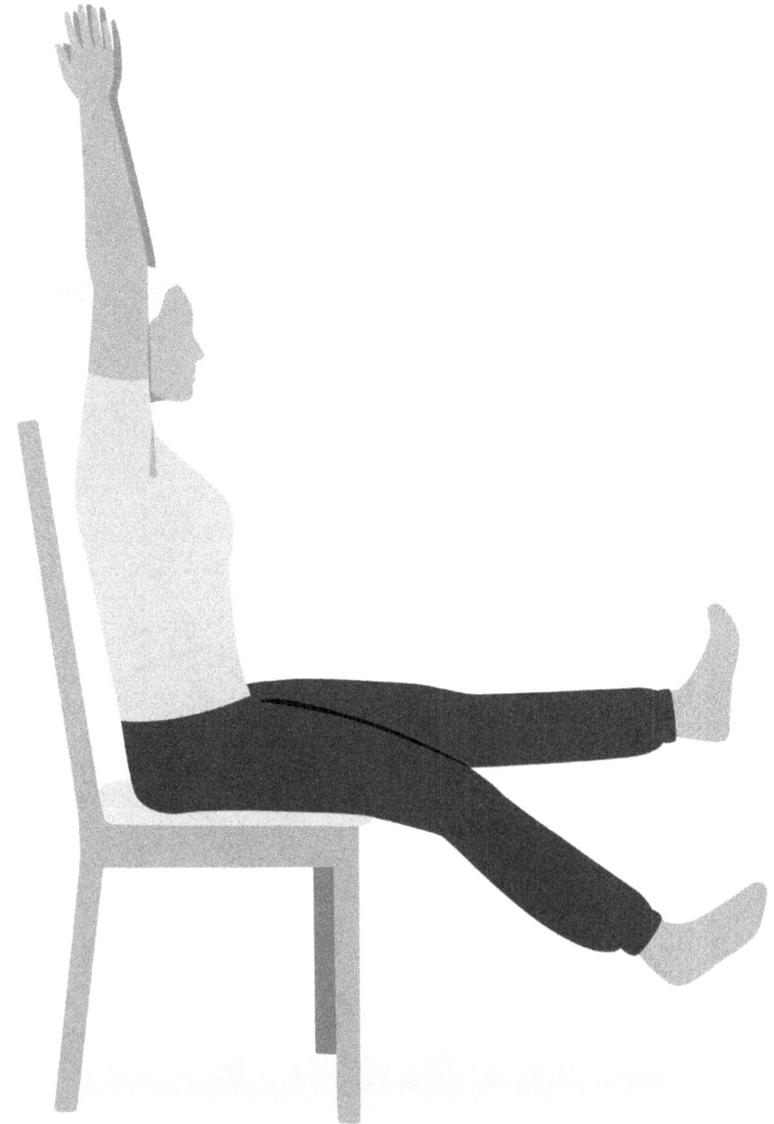

Lower Body Strength: Leg and Hip Exercises

Sit to Stand

1. Start your practice by sitting upright toward the front of your chair and relaxing your neck and shoulders. Your feet should be flat on the floor, about hip-width apart, with your knees in line with your ankles. Your hands can be resting on your thighs.

2. Move your feet backward so that your heels are now positioned behind your knees.

3. Lean forward from your hips so you bring your nose in front of your toes. You can place your hands on the chair, armrests, or your thighs for support.

4. Stand up and keep equal weight on both legs and feet.

5. Make sure your legs are fully extended at the hips and knees when you stand.

6. Sit down by pushing your hips backward, reaching for the chair, and sitting down.

7. Repeat for as many repetitions as required.

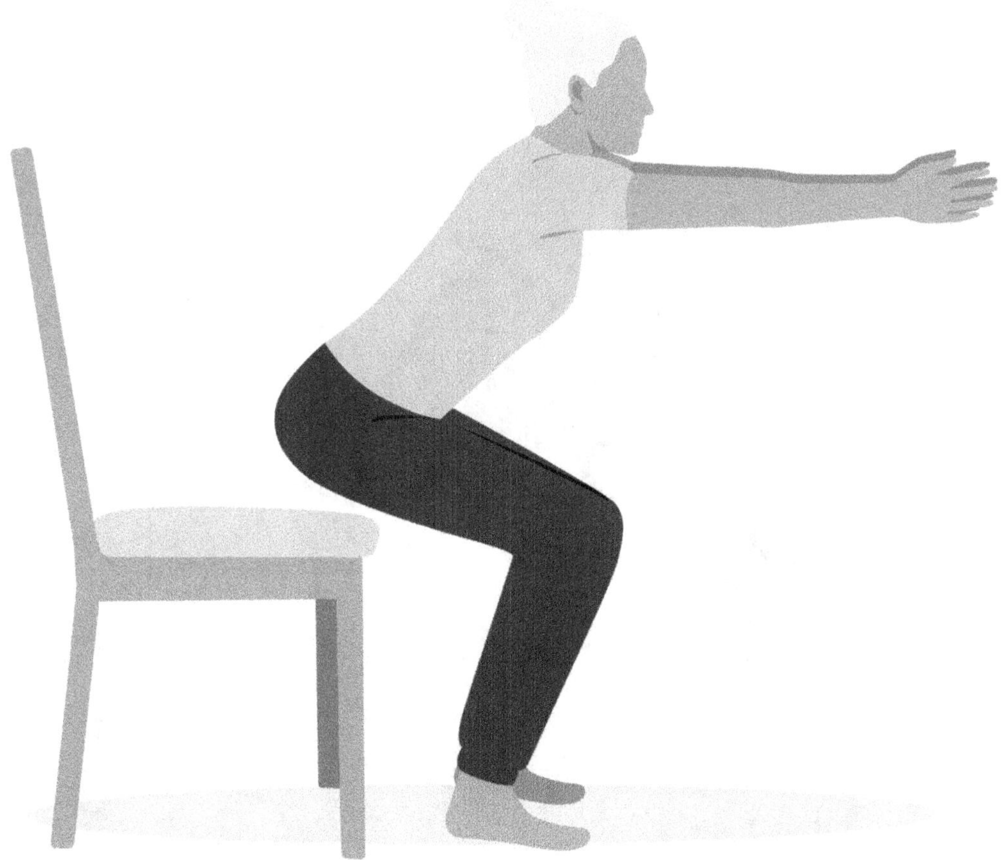

Seated Hip Flexions

1. Start your practice by sitting upright toward the front of your chair and relaxing your neck and shoulders. Your feet should be flat on the floor, about hip-width apart, with your knees in line with your ankles. Your hands can be resting on your thighs.

2. Slowly lift your right foot off the floor, bending your knee and bringing it toward your chest.

3. Hold your right knee in the bent position for a few seconds, feeling the stretch in your hamstrings.

4. Gently lower your right foot back down to the floor.

5. Repeat the same steps with your left foot, lifting it off the floor and bringing it toward your chest for a stretch.

6. Alternate between your right and left legs for as many repetitions as required.

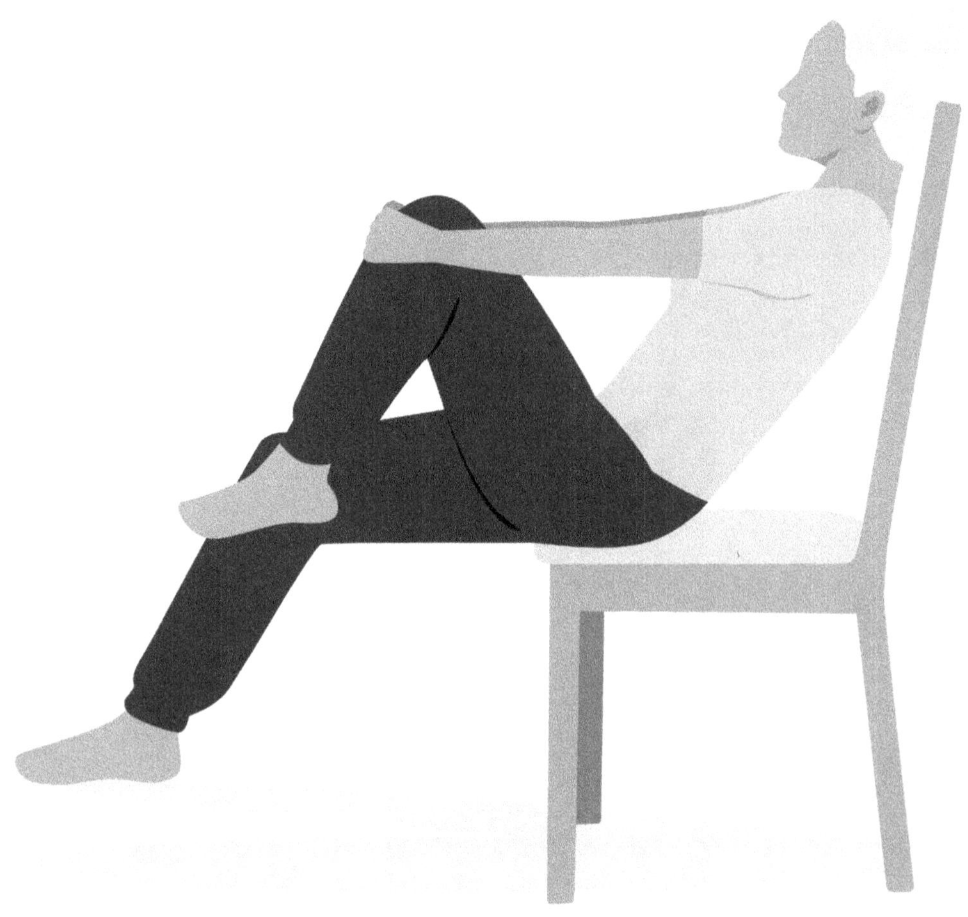

Seated Hip Abductions

1. Start your practice by sitting upright toward the front of your chair and relaxing your neck and shoulders. Your feet should be flat on the floor, about hip-width apart, with your knees in line with your ankles. Your hands can be resting on your thighs.

2. Place your hands on the outside of your knees.

3. Create resistance by using your knees to push against your hands. Resist the outward force of your knees created by your hands. (Optional: use resistance band)

4. Hold this position for five seconds and relax.

5. Repeat for as many repetitions as required.

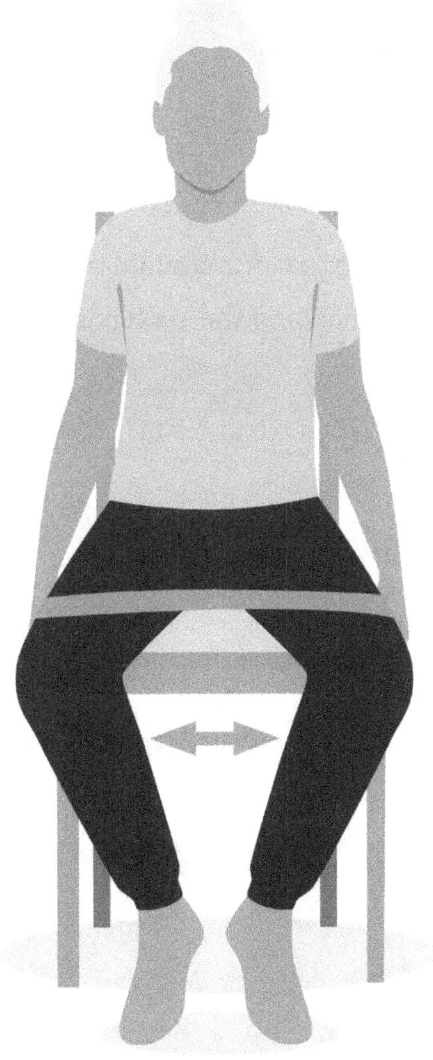

Balance Exercises

Our ability to maintain balance declines with age, increasing our risk of falls and injury. Maintaining and improving our balance is crucial for a safe and independent lifestyle. Chair yoga is an effective way to enhance balance.

Balance begins to decline after the age of 40, and this decline accelerates with age. One of the main causes of injuries among the elderly is falls, and one major contributing factor to falls is poor balance. By incorporating balance-focused exercises, such as those found in chair yoga, we can significantly reduce our risk of falls.

Apart from reducing the risk of falls, improving balance has a range of other benefits, such as:

- Enhancing coordination and mobility

- Increasing confidence in daily activities

- Promoting better posture

- Supporting overall physical independence

Seniors who regularly practice chair yoga can maintain and enhance their balance, leading to a safer and more active lifestyle. Start practicing these exercises for improved balance.

Single Leg Balance

1. Begin by standing upright in back of your chair, with the back facing you. Relax your shoulders and your neck. Keep your feet about hip-width apart.

2. Carefully raise your left leg by bending at the knee to hip height and holding it a few inches above the chair seat, or if you cannot manage that, place it on the chair for support. Keep as much weight off it as possible, as all of your weight should be on your right standing leg.

3. Raise your arms to chest level so they are parallel to the ground. If this is easy for you, you can raise your arms overhead.

4. Hold for as long as required.

5. Lower your leg and your arms.

6. Swap sides and repeat.

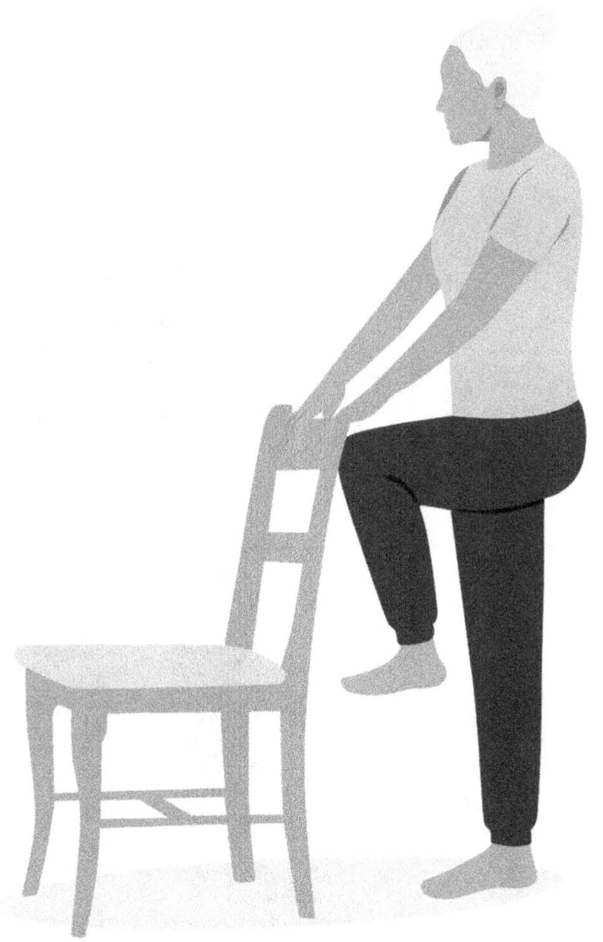

Extended Leg Balance

1. Begin by standing upright in back of your chair, with the back facing you. Relax your shoulders and your neck. Keep your feet about hip-width apart.

2. Carefully raise your left leg by bending at the knee to hip height and holding it a few inches above the chair seat.

3. Slowly and carefully extend your left leg out behind you as you hinge forward from your waist and rest your hands on the seat.

4. Lift your leg as high as you can, elongating it behind you as far as you feel comfortable while still maintaining your balance.

5. Hold for as long as required.

6. Lower your leg and come back up to a standing position.

7. Swap sides and repeat with the other leg.

8. Alternate for as many repetitions as required.

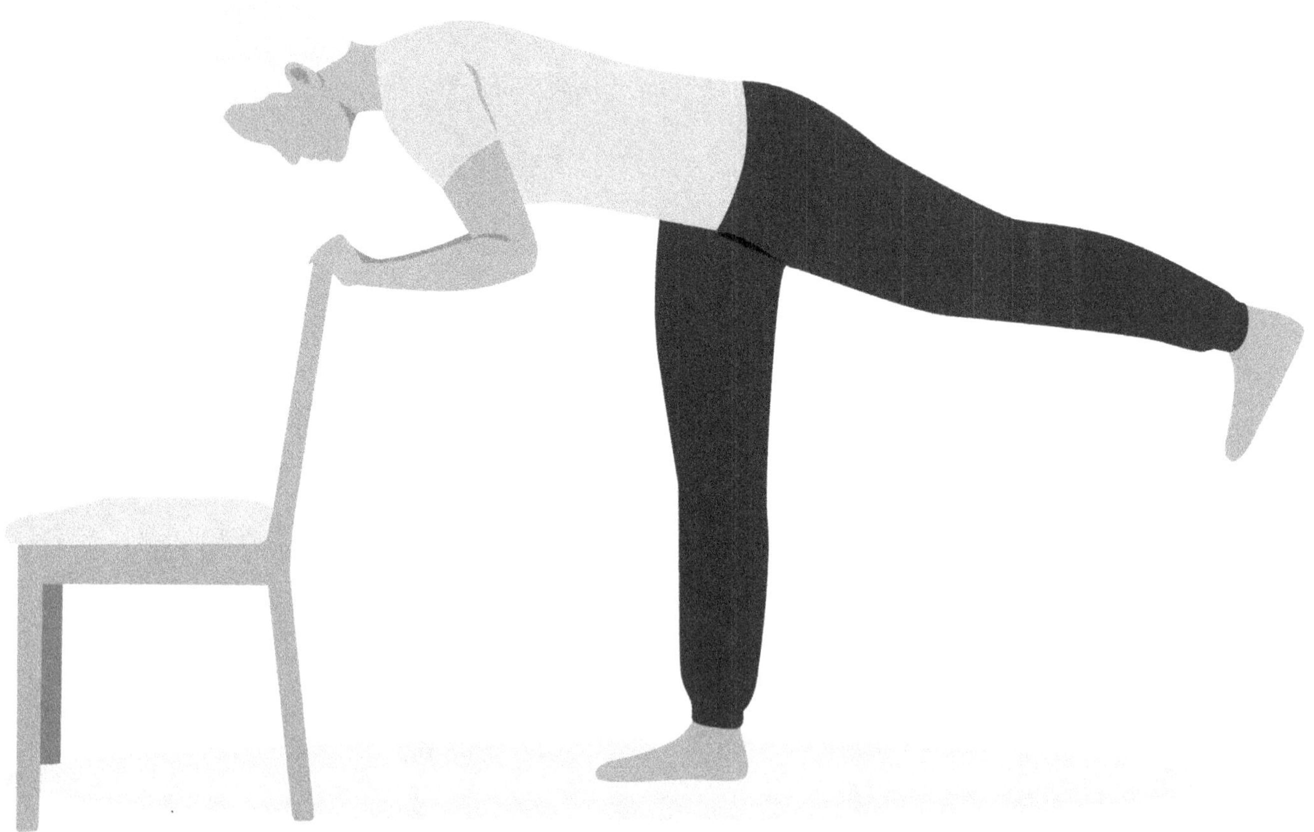

Chair Bird Dog

1. Begin by standing upright in front of your chair, with the seat facing you. Relax your shoulders and your neck. Keep your feet about hip-width apart.

2. Folding forward from your hips, bend over and put your hands on the seat of your chair.

3. Slowly and carefully extend your left leg out behind you and simultaneously raise your right arm out in front of you. Hold for one breath.

4. Release by lowering your arm and leg.

5. Swap sides and repeat on your right leg and left arm.

6. Alternate for as many repetitions as required.

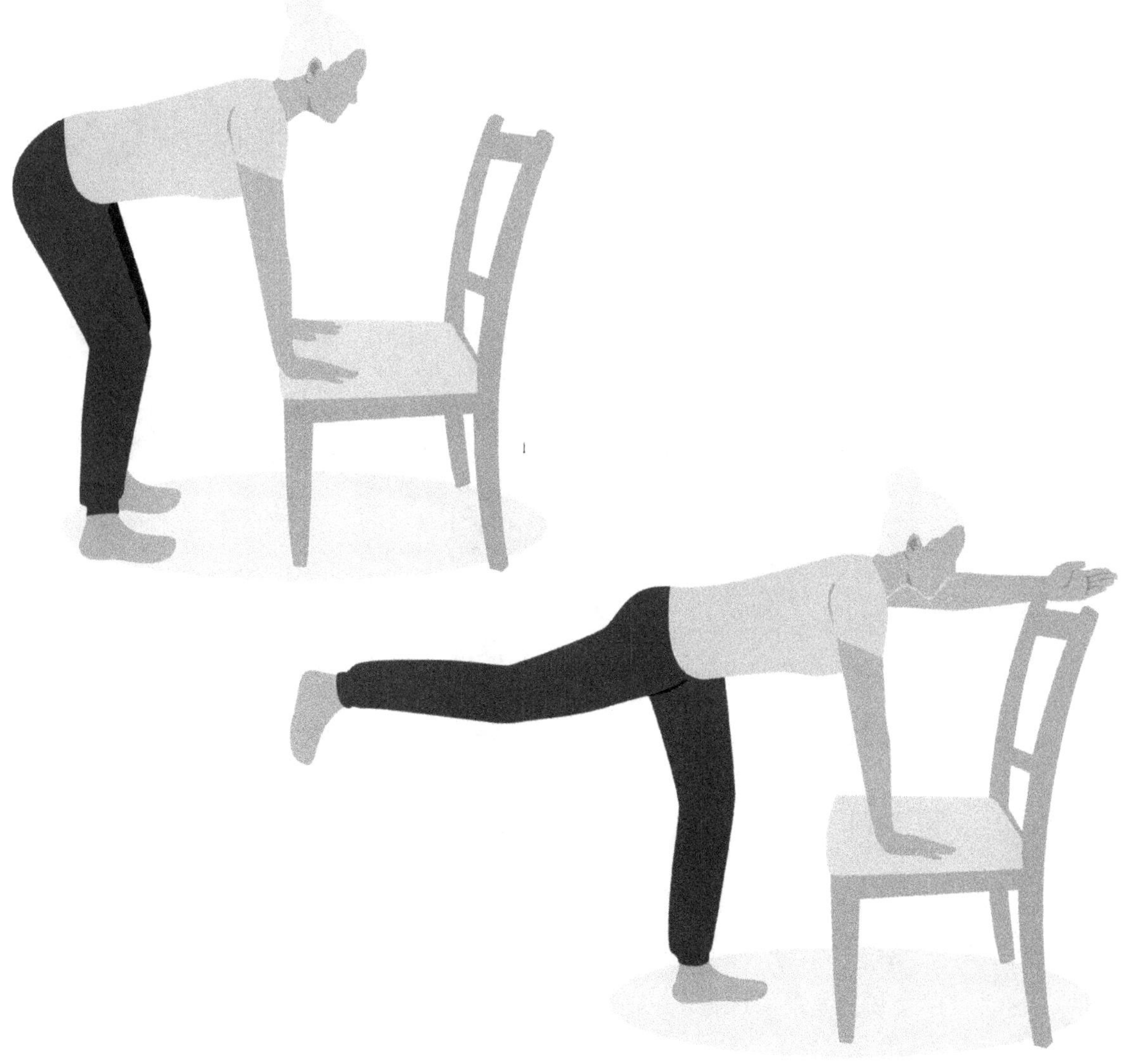

Half Moon Pose

1. Begin by standing upright next to your chair. Relax your shoulders and your neck. Keep your feet about hip-width apart.

2. Take a wide-legged stance, with the toes of your feet closest to the chair pointing out toward it. Your other foot should be turned in slightly.

3. Carefully reach for the seat of the chair while raising your back leg. Release and come back to standing.

4. Repeat for as many repetitions as required.

5. Swap sides and repeat on the other leg.

6. Repeat for as many repetitions as required.

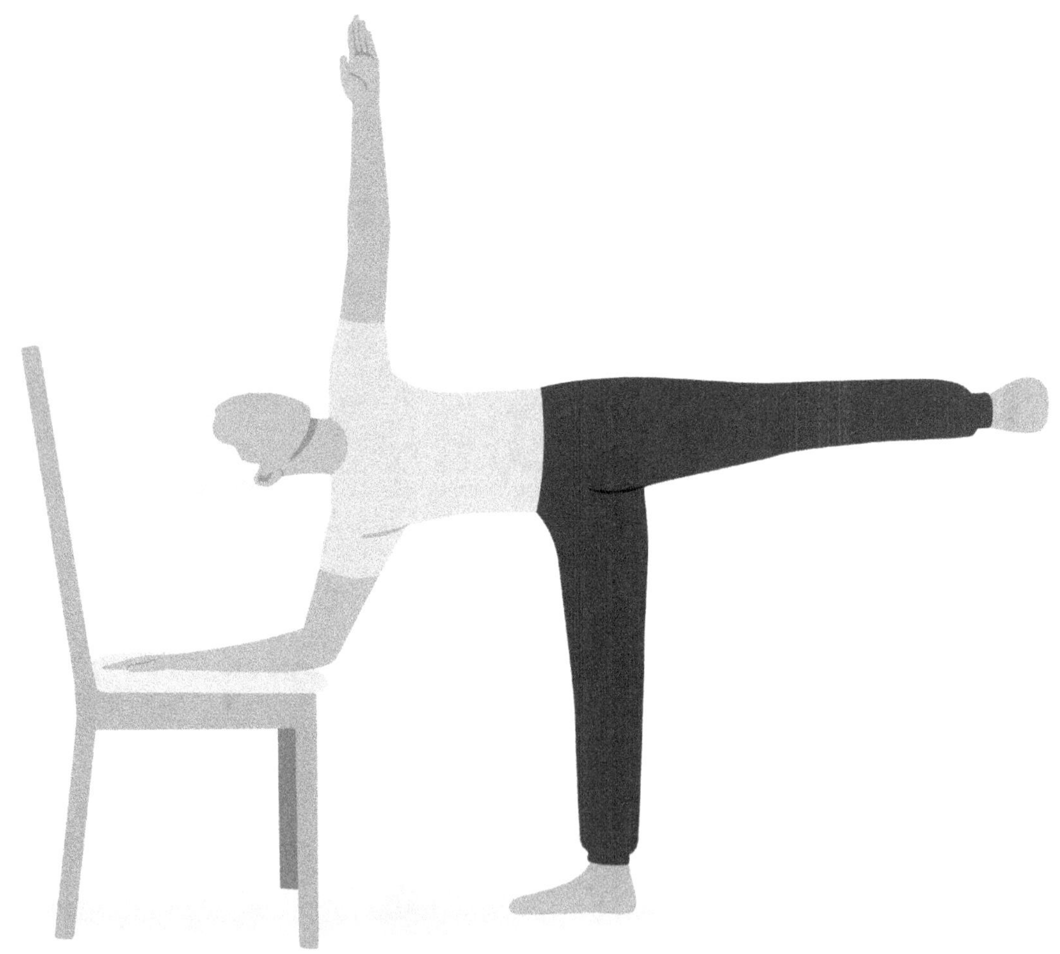

Combinations for Comprehensive Care

The CDC advises that adults over 50 should aim to perform 150 minutes of moderate-intensity exercise a week, as well as two days of strengthening activities. For those of us 65 years and older, we should add activities that improve balance as well (CDC, 2023).

You can use a combination of the above exercises to create a strength routine to perform twice a week. Begin each workout with some simple warm-up routines and add in one or two stretches. Do the same when you cool down; this is the perfect time to stretch out your muscles and help initiate your recovery.

A good session would look like the following:

1. warm-up routine

2. stretching

3. flow

4. cool-down routine

Here is an example:

Warm-Up:

1. Start your practice by sitting upright in your chair and relaxing your neck and shoulders. Your feet should be flat on the floor, about hip-width apart, with your knees in line with your ankles. Your hands can be resting on your thighs.

2. Gently bring your right ear to your right shoulder, and rotate your head in a clockwise direction.

3. Rotate for 12 repetitions.

4. Relax and switch directions.

5. Raise your arms out to your sides, in line with your shoulders.

6. Keeping your arms straight and moving from your shoulders, gently rotate your arms forward.

7. Start with small circles, and as you progress, let them get bigger.

8. Repeat for 10-15 repetitions.

9. Relax and repeat in the other direction.

10. Cross your arms in front of your chest.

11. Rotate your upper body to the left for as far as you feel comfortable and hold for as long as needed.

12. Return to a neutral position.

13. Rotate your upper body to the right for as far as you feel comfortable and hold for as long as needed.

14. Extend your left leg out in front of you. Keep it straight and point your toes toward the ceiling.

15. Keep your back straight and your chest upright as you gently fold forward from your hips.

16. Hold for 15 seconds.

17. Swap legs and repeat.

Stretches

1. Start your practice by sitting upright in your chair and relaxing your neck and shoulders. Your feet should be flat on the floor, about hip-width apart, with your knees in line with your ankles. Your hands can be resting on your thighs.

2. Raise your left arm overhead, keeping it in line with your ears.

3. Reach to the right, keeping your torso facing forward.

4. Hold for 30 seconds.

5. Swap arms and repeat.

6. Extend your left leg out in front of you, keeping your right bent at the knee.

7. Bend forward from your hips and carefully slide your hands down your left leg as you feel a stretch in your hamstring. Extend as far as you feel comfortable.

8. Hold for 30 seconds.

9. Swap sides and repeat on your right side.

Flow

1. Start your practice by sitting upright in your chair and relaxing your neck and shoulders. Your feet should be flat on the floor, about hip-width apart, with your knees in line with your ankles. Your hands can be resting on your thighs.

2. Elongate your spine by raising your chest and dropping your shoulders.

3. Take a deep breath in through your nose and close your eyes; your air should expand into your belly.

4. Breathe out slowly through your mouth while focusing on releasing tension.

5. Keep your breath even as you ground yourself by imagining that roots are growing into the ground from your feet.

6. Stay here for a minute.

7. Turn your body to the right and move your buttocks closer to the left edge of the chair. This will create support for your right thigh.

8. Stretch your left leg behind you and straighten it out as much as possible. Place the ball of your foot on the floor, keeping your heel lifted. Bend your left knee at a 90-degree angle, keeping it aligned with your ankle.

9. Raise your arms above you, reaching to the ceiling with your palms facing each other. Alternatively, put your hands on your hips or the seat of the chair for support.

10. Keep your chest raised, and relax your shoulders. Keep your gaze forward.

11. Hold this pose for a minute, then release and swap sides.

12. Breathe in and arch your back while looking up at the ceiling.

13. Breathe in and out deeply as you hold for as long as needed.

14. When you are ready to release, breathe out and slowly roll your head up to a neutral position.

15. Breathe in as you lengthen your spine, and as you breathe out, twist to the right.

16. Put your right hand on the chair's back and your left hand on the outside of your right thigh.

17. Keep your spine long and twist from your torso, not just from your shoulders.

18. Look over your right shoulder for a deeper twist.

19. Hold the twist for 30 seconds.

20. Inhale to release the twist back to the center.

21. Repeat the twist on the other side by twisting to the left.

22. Place both your hands behind your head, with your elbows facing out to the side.

23. Gently rotate your upper body and bring your left elbow gently across your body to the right.

24. Lift your right leg up simultaneously, keeping the knee bent.

25. Release and return to the center.

26. Gently rotate your upper body and bring your right elbow gently across your body to the left.

27. Lift your left leg up simultaneously, keeping the knee bent.

28. Repeat for 12 repetitions.

Cool-Down Sequence

1. Start your practice by sitting upright in your chair and relaxing your neck and shoulders. Your feet should be flat on the floor, about hip-width apart, with your knees in line with your ankles. Your hands can be resting on your thighs.

2. Bring your palms together in front of your chest in a prayer position. Breathe in and out.

3. As you breathe in again, lift the arms over your head, look up, and bend back slightly.

4. Breathe out and bend forward.

5. Wrap your hands around your left shin. If this is uncomfortable, wrap your hands under your knee or thigh.

6. Breathe in and lift the left leg from the ground toward the chest, with the knee bent.

7. Breathe out and release your left leg back down.

8. Breathe in and bring your upper body back to your neutral position.

9. Raise your arms above your head.

10. Breathe out and bend forward.

11. Wrap your hands around your right shin. If this is uncomfortable, wrap your hands under your knee or thigh.

12. Breathe in and lift the right leg from the ground toward the chest, with the knee bent.

13. Breathe out and release your left leg back down, and let your arms hang at your side.

14. Breathe in and circle your left arm up toward the right to lengthen the left side of your body. Your eyes should follow your hand.

15. Breathe out and release the arm back down.

16. Breathe in and circle your right arm up toward the left to lengthen your right side of the body. Your eyes should follow your hand.

17. Breathe out and return your arm to the outside of your left knee.

18. Breathe in and open your left arm to the left, parallel to the ground. Look over your left shoulder.

19. Breathe out and return to the center.

20. Place your left hand on the outside of your right knee.

21. Inhale, extend your right arm to the right, rotating with your spine straight.

22. Breathe out and return to the center.

23. Breathe in, lean forward, and place your elbows on your thighs. Arch your back while raising your chest and looking upward.

24. Breathe out and release.

25. Breathe in to rise back up to a seated position with arms overhead.

Stretching

1. Start your practice by sitting upright in your chair and relaxing your neck and shoulders. Your feet should be flat on the floor, about hip-width apart, with your knees in line with your ankles. Your hands can be resting on your thighs.

2. Raise both of your arms straight in front of you at shoulder height.

3. Arch your back and lower your head in between your arms as you keep them straight.

4. Hold this position for two breaths. Release to neutral position.

5. Repeat for eight repetitions.

6. Stretch your legs so that they are slightly in front of your chair.

7. Lean back against your chair.

8. Lift your left leg up, bending at the knee, and take hold of it at the knee with both of your hands.

9. Hug your left knee by pulling it to your chest.

10. Hold for 30 seconds.

11. Swap legs and repeat on the right side.

All these poses can be modified based on your needs. As we mentioned in the previous chapters, this can be done by modifying the poses using different props such as blocks or straps.

Safeguarding Progress

Now that you have the tools to start your practice, how can you incorporate it into your daily life and make sure that you remain consistent?

You need to build it into a habit. The important thing to remember here, which is often overlooked by those with an all-or-nothing mindset, is that we are aiming for progress and not perfection. We want to be consistent, as consistency brings results.

How do we do this? We will draw from some of the advice that James Clear provides. The first thing to do is to begin small. I know that you are excited and highly motivated to start your fitness journey, and while I encourage you to use this drive, you do not need to go all in.

You are more likely to be and stay successful if you start off small. Clear advises that you pick a task that is so manageable you can do it even when you are unmotivated and your willpower has waned. An example could be that you just sit on your chair and do six cat-cow poses (Clear, 2014).

This should take you less than two minutes, which follows his "two-minute rule." This rule focuses on just starting your workout for two minutes and not worrying about whether you will continue or not; if you do two minutes, your day has been a success. More often than not, these two minutes end up extending and you finish your workout.

To develop a habit, you need to repeat an action over and over, which means you just need to start.

But what if you have difficulty starting? Well, apart from the two-minute rule and making your habit simple, you could also set a schedule for yourself. Think of it as setting a meeting that you cannot miss.

You can use this as a template:

"During the week, I will do a chair yoga session on [DAY] at [TIME OF DAY] at/in [PLACE]."

Finally, the last tip is to focus on the habit and not the outcome. For example, when it comes to exercising, you may hear people talking about how they want to lose five pounds. This places the focus on the goal and not the system, but in the beginning, your focus needs to be on how you reach your goal, not the goal itself. In the beginning, you want to be a person who practices chair yoga regularly, and that should be your main focus.

Once you become a person that does chair yoga every week, you can shift your focus to improving other areas of your practice, because "without the habit, strategy is useless" (Clear, 2014).

Overcoming Plateaus

So what happens when we reach a plateau and we fall off the exercise wagon? Better yet, how do we prevent this from happening? Here are some tips to keep you on your chair.

It Is Not All-Or-Nothing

Some activity is always better than no activity. We often get into an all-or-nothing mindset, where if something has thrown us off our plans, we tend to ditch them entirely. It is okay if your plans are derailed. Do what you can and move on; tomorrow is another day.

Find Your "Why"

If we look deeper, we will find motivation for our actions that are often more than just "losing weight" or "getting fit." It is this deeper reason that will keep us motivated and determined on days when we would rather throw in the towel.

I like to use the "5 Whys" exercise, which is a problem-solving exercise that has been modified by Precision Nutrition to be used by those looking to find their deep motivation (Precision Nutrition, n.d.).

First, ask yourself why you want to accomplish something. Then you go on to question yourself a further four times to find the root of your reasons. Here is an example:

"Why are you starting chair yoga?"

"I want to maintain my fitness."

"Why do you want to maintain your fitness?"

"Because I am getting older, and I feel a decline as I age."

"Why is that important to you?"

"Because I need to maintain fitness to continue to do the things I love."

"Why does that matter?"

"Because I have grandchildren that I want to continue to be active with as long as I can."

As you can see, we manage to get to the bigger picture and motivation that fuels our goal. The goal of maintaining a healthy lifestyle so that you can continue to be a significant part of your grandchildren's lives is far more motivating than just trying to stay fit, right?

Set Goals That Are Right For You

Whether you have been in fitness for a long time or are just starting out, you need to set goals that meet you where you are. In most instances, this means setting small and challenging goals that are also achievable. This ensures that you are constantly moving forward and making progress while also keeping you motivated with achievements.

Track Your Progress

Keep track of all your measures of success, not only the ones related to goals. Track how you feel, your energy levels, your mood, or even your eating habits. These are all victories that indicate you are moving forward and in the correct direction.

And when you do see progress, reward yourself for your efforts. It does not have to cost anything either; you could simply reward yourself by binge-watching your favorite show!

Be Patient and Practice Compassion

Success does not happen overnight, and it often takes weeks or months to establish a habit. There are certainly times when you may hit a speed bump or two and your progress stalls.

This is where our all-or-nothing mindset shift comes into play and we allow ourselves to do the best we can, even if it looks different to the plans we had set. Life happens, and when it does, we need to allow ourselves some wiggle room without guilt.

Take a moment to relax and engage in self-compassion exercises. Never forget that you are your own greatest supporter.

Key Takeaways

- Flexibility is essential for you to maintain healthy movement patterns and reduce the risk of injury.

- Strength training can help combat muscle loss with aging and improve overall physical well-being.

- A combination of moderate-intensity exercise, strengthening activities, and balance improvement exercises is recommended for all healthy individuals.

- Starting small, setting achievable goals, tracking progress, and practicing self-compassion can help you establish a consistent exercise routine.

- Consistency is key in maintaining physical fitness and overall well-being as you get older.

CHAPTER 6

Focused Practices for Specific Needs

The beauty of chair yoga is that it can be adapted for anyone, and many people may find that they need to modify certain movements to accommodate their needs. Some instances where modification would be needed are if you suffer from arthritis or osteoporosis.

This chapter will provide the movements best suited to help chronic pain, arthritis, and back pain.

Understanding Arthritis and Osteoporosis

Bone health is crucial as we age, especially since our bodies start losing muscle mass and bone density the older we get. Typically, around the age of 35, the body's ability to replace lost bone decreases, leading to conditions like osteoporosis (Sullivan Barger, 2022). This decrease in bone density can make bones weaker and more prone to fractures, with the backbone being particularly at risk. Vertebral compression fractures are a common risk associated with weak bones (Sullivan Barger, 2022).

Importance of Yoga for Bone Health

Engaging in activities like yoga can be beneficial for promoting better bone health. Several research investigations have demonstrated the beneficial effects of yoga, as it acts to stimulate the body to generate more bone tissue. Through regular yoga practice, you can strengthen your bones, resulting in a reduced risk of fractures and injuries. Not only does this activity improve bone health, but it also improves physical wellness in general.

Yoga is a holistic method of building bone density by integrating physical postures, breathing exercises, and relaxation techniques. Some yoga positions require you to bear some weight, which helps strengthen your skeleton and promote bone development. Additionally, the mindfulness aspect of yoga promotes mental well-being, which is integral to maintaining overall health and vitality as we age.

Yoga is an excellent way to improve bone health and guard against fractures and osteoporosis. With specific yoga poses and mindful movements, you can strengthen your bones, improve balance, and protect against potential injuries.

Chronic Pain Management

Working through chronic pain can be tough. Yoga can provide relief for those dealing with this discomfort.

But yoga doesn't just stop at alleviating physical discomfort. It goes a step further and addresses the mental challenges that come with long-term suffering. This practice not only helps calm your mind but also teaches you tools to better cope with the emotional toll that chronic pain can take on your mental health. This is why many health professionals recommend yoga for chronic pain— it offers a holistic approach to healing. Yoga addresses mental and emotional well-being in addition to physical issues.

Your body and mind start to become more deeply connected as a result of yoga practice. As you stretch and breathe, you become more attuned to the signals your body sends you, allowing you to respond to your physical and emotional needs more effectively. This newfound awareness can be empowering, helping you regain a sense of control over your body despite the chronic pain.

Tips for Practicing Chair Yoga with Pain

- Breathe Deeply: Focus on deep, mindful breathing to enhance relaxation and pain relief.

- Move Slowly: Perform movements slowly and gently to avoid strain.

- Modify Poses: Adjust poses to fit your comfort level and range of motion.

- Consult a Professional: Work with a certified yoga instructor or physical therapist to ensure exercises are appropriate for your condition.

Chair yoga can be particularly effective for addressing common pain areas in seniors. Here are some of the most common pain areas and how chair yoga can help:

Common Pain Areas for Seniors and Chair Yoga Solutions

Lower Back Pain

Chair Downward-Facing Dog Helps with Lower Back Pain by:

- Stretching: Stretches the lower back muscles and elongates the spine to ease stiffness and tension.

- Decompressing: Relieves pressure on the lumbar spine by encouraging proper alignment and elongation of the vertebrae.

- Improving Flexibility: Enhances the flexibility of the lower back and hamstrings, which can alleviate strain on the lower back.

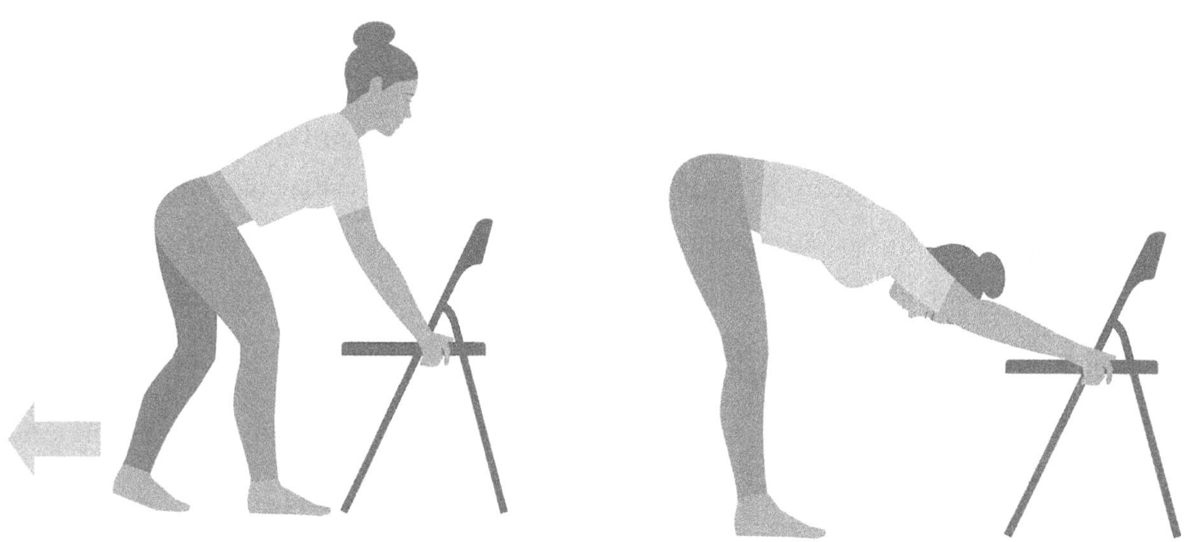

1. Start your practice by standing in front of your chair. Relax your neck and shoulders. Your feet should be hip-width apart.

2. Place your hands on the seat of your chair and carefully walk your feet backward until your body is at a 45-degree angle to the floor.

3. Breathe in and activate your midline muscles; your lower back and hips should be raised and your head and shoulders relaxed.

4. Hold this pose for as long as needed, and when you are ready to release, walk your feet back toward the chair and stand up.

Seated Twist Helps with Lower Back Pain by:

- Stretching: Gently stretches the muscles and soft tissues around the lumbar spine, relieving tightness and tension.

- Increasing Mobility: Enhances spinal flexibility and range of motion, reducing stiffness in the lower back.

- Releasing Tension: Alleviates built-up tension in the lower back and surrounding muscles, which can help reduce pain.

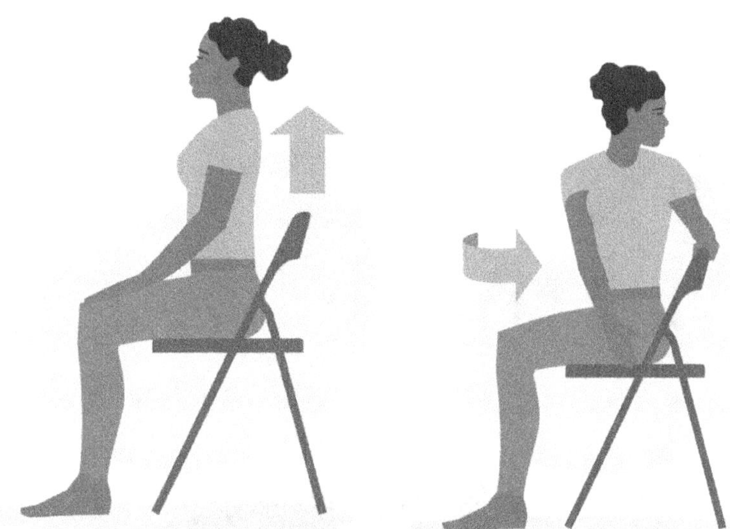

1. Start your practice by sitting upright in your chair and relaxing your neck and shoulders. Your feet should be flat on the floor, about hip-width apart, with your knees in line with your ankles. Your hands can be resting on your thighs.

2. Breathe in as you lengthen your spine, and as you breathe out, twist to the right.

3. Put your right hand on the chair's back and your left hand on the outside of your right thigh.

4. Keep your spine long and twist from your torso, not just from your shoulders.

5. Look over your right shoulder for a deeper twist.

6. Hold the twist for as long as needed.

7. Inhale to release the twist back to the center.

8. Repeat the twist on the other side by twisting to the left.

Lumbar Extensions Directly Targets Lower Back Pain by:

- Stretching: Elongates and loosens tight lower back muscles, reducing stiffness.

- Strengthening: Fortifies the muscles that support the lumbar spine, enhancing stability.

- Improving Posture: Promotes better spinal alignment, alleviating pressure on the lower back.

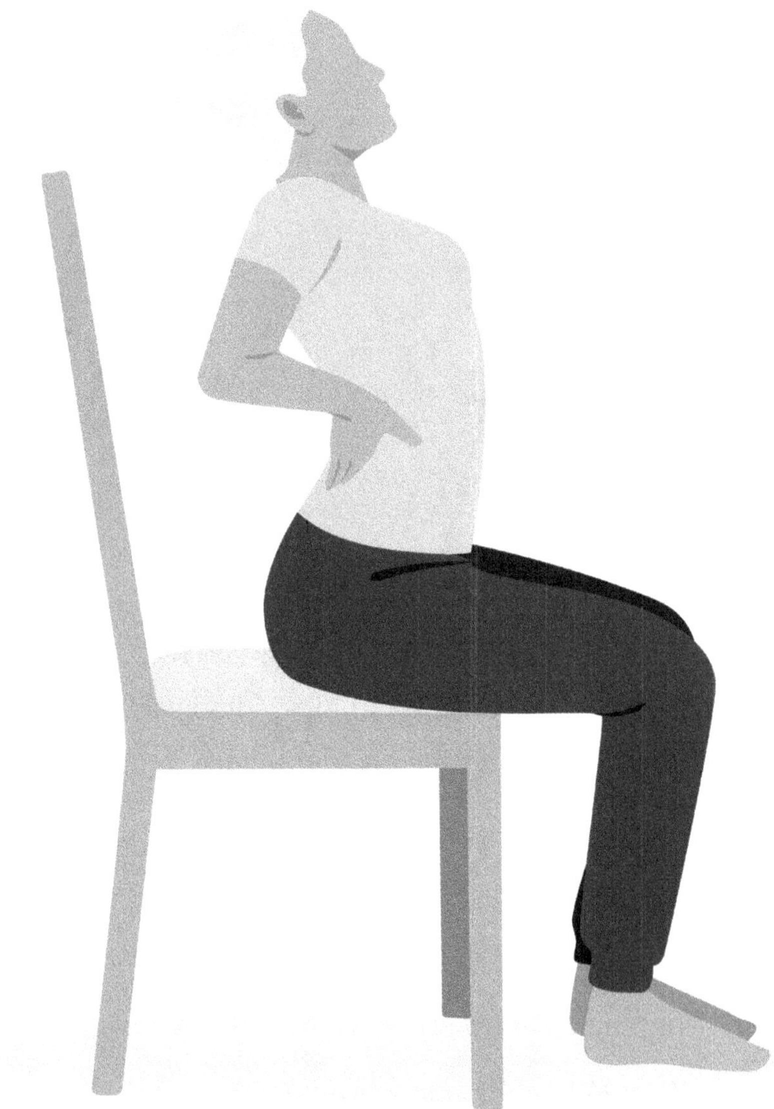

1. Start your practice by sitting upright in your chair and relaxing your neck and shoulders. Your feet should be flat on the floor, about hip-width apart, with your knees in line with your ankles. Your hands can be resting on your thighs.

2. Place your hands on the bottom of your back.

3. Gently lean back into your hands and slightly arch your back.

4. Hold for as long as needed.

Torso Rotations Specifically Target Lower Back Pain by:

- Stretching: They help stretch the muscles and tissues around the lumbar spine.

- Improving Flexibility: Enhancing spinal flexibility can alleviate stiffness and discomfort.

- Relieving Tension: Rotating the torso helps to release tension and reduce muscle tightness in the lower back.

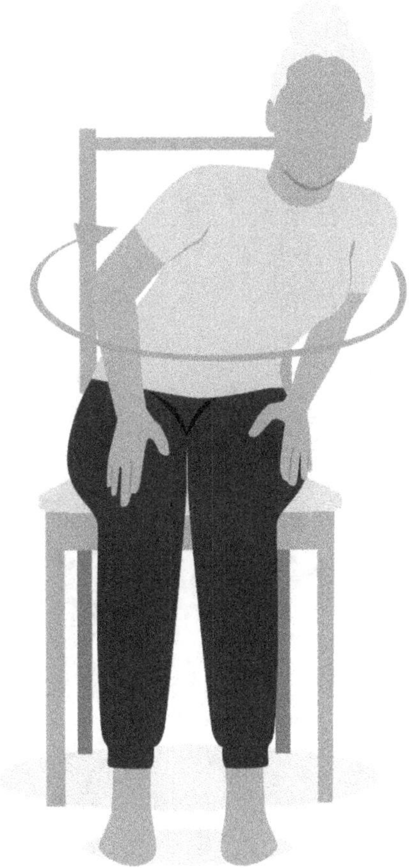

1. Start your practice by sitting upright in your chair and relaxing your neck and shoulders. Your feet should be flat on the floor, about hip-width apart, with your knees in line with your ankles. Your hands can be resting on your thighs.

2. Breathe in and begin rotating your torso in large, gentle circles in a clockwise direction.

3. Allow your head and neck to follow the movement of your torso.

4. Continue the circular motion for as long as required.

5. Switch directions and repeat the circular motion in the opposite direction.

Hip Pain

Hip Flexions Help Hip Pain by:

- Stretching: Relieves tightness in the hip flexor muscles, which can be a source of hip pain.

- Improving Mobility: Reduces stiffness and pain by expanding the hip joint's range of motion.

- Alleviating Pressure: Improves muscular balance and flexibility, which lessens stress on the hip joint.

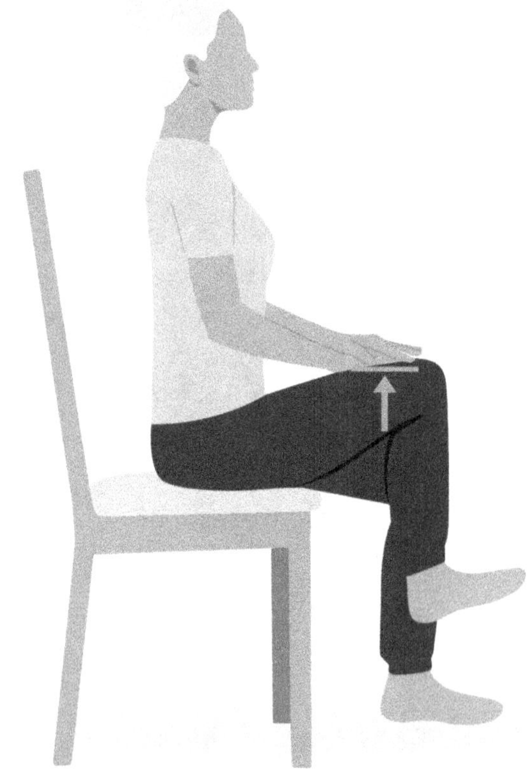

1. Start your practice by sitting upright in your chair and relaxing your neck and shoulders. Your feet should be flat on the floor, about hip-width apart, with your knees in line with your ankles. Your hands can be resting on your thighs.

2. Lift your left leg, keeping your knee bent.

3. Hold for one breath and gently lower it back to the ground.

4. Repeat for as many reps as needed.

5. Swap sides and repeat.

Chair Warrior One & Two Helps with Hip Pain by

- Stretching: Extends and loosens tight hip flexor muscles, alleviating tension and discomfort.

- Strengthening: Builds strength in the hip muscles, providing better support and reducing strain on the hip joint.

- Improving Alignment: Promotes proper hip alignment, which can reduce uneven pressure and alleviate pain.

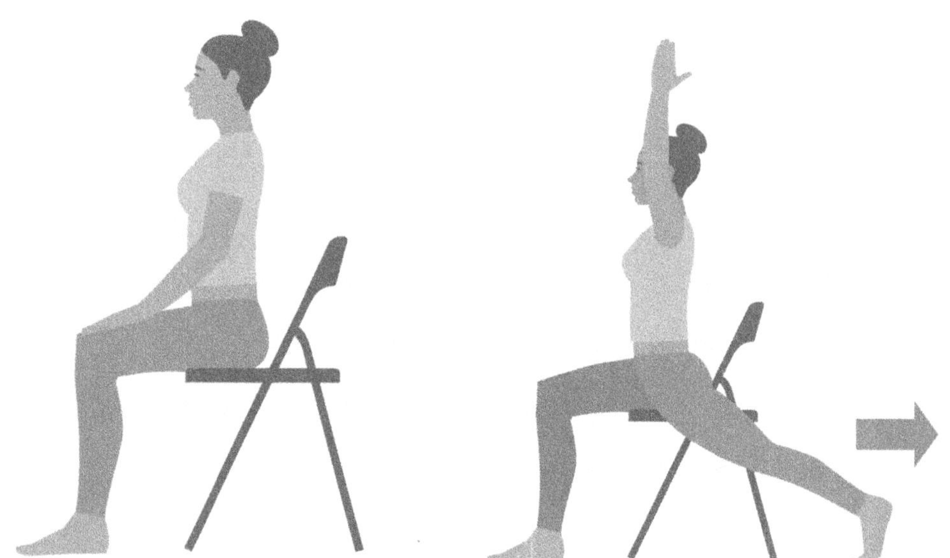

1. Start your practice by sitting upright toward the front of your chair and relaxing your neck and shoulders. Your feet should be flat on the floor, about hip-width apart, with your knees in line with your ankles. Your hands can be resting on your thighs.

2. Turn your body to the right and move your buttocks closer to the left edge of the chair. This will create support for your right thigh.

3. Stretch your left leg behind you and straighten it out as much as possible. Place the ball of your foot on the floor, keeping your heel lifted. Bend your left knee at a 90-degree angle, keeping it aligned with your ankle.

4. Raise your arms above you, reaching to the ceiling, with your palms facing each other. Alternatively, put your hands on your hips or the seat of the chair for support.

5. Keep your chest raised, and relax your shoulders. Keep your gaze forward.

6. Hold this pose for as long as needed, then release and swap sides.

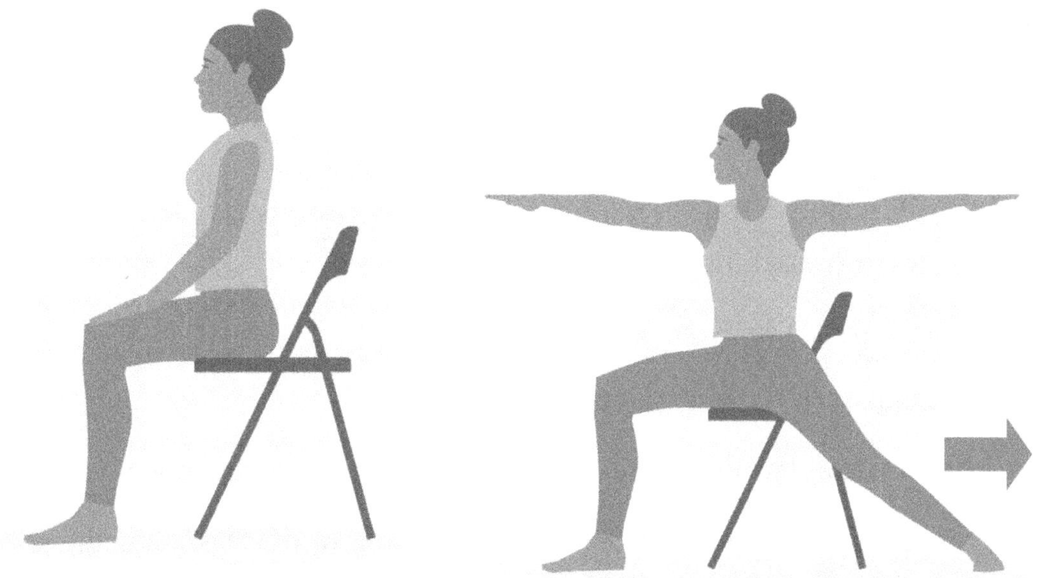

1. Start your practice by sitting upright toward the front of your chair and relaxing your neck and shoulders. Your feet should be flat on the floor, about hip-width apart, with your knees in line with your ankles. Your hands can be resting on your thighs.

2. Turn your body to the right and move your buttocks closer to the left edge of the chair. This will create support for your right thigh.

3. Stretch your left leg behind you and straighten it out as much as possible. Place the ball of your foot on the floor, keeping your heel lifted. Bend your left knee at a 90-degree angle, keeping it aligned with your ankle.

4. Raise your arms out to the sides at shoulder height, palms facing down, in a T-position.

5. Gaze over your left hand.

6. Keep your shoulders relaxed and your spine elongated.

7. Hold this pose for as long as needed, then release and swap sides.

Knee Pain

Chair Warrior One & Two (Exercises above) Also Help with Knee Pain by:

- Strengthening: Strengthens and engages the knee-supporting muscles, giving the joint more stability and support.

- Improving Alignment: Promotes proper knee alignment, which can reduce uneven pressure and strain on the knee joint.

- Enhancing Flexibility: Improves range of motion and lessens stiffness in the knee by stretching the surrounding muscles and ligaments.

(See Chair Warrior One & Two Exercises above)

Seated Toe Touches Help with Knee Pain by:

- Stretching: Releases tension in the calf and hamstring muscles, reducing knee joint strain.

- Improving Flexibility: Enhances the range of motion in the legs, reducing stiffness in the knees.

- Relieving Tension: Eases the tightness in the muscles surrounding the knee, which lessens pain and improves mobility.

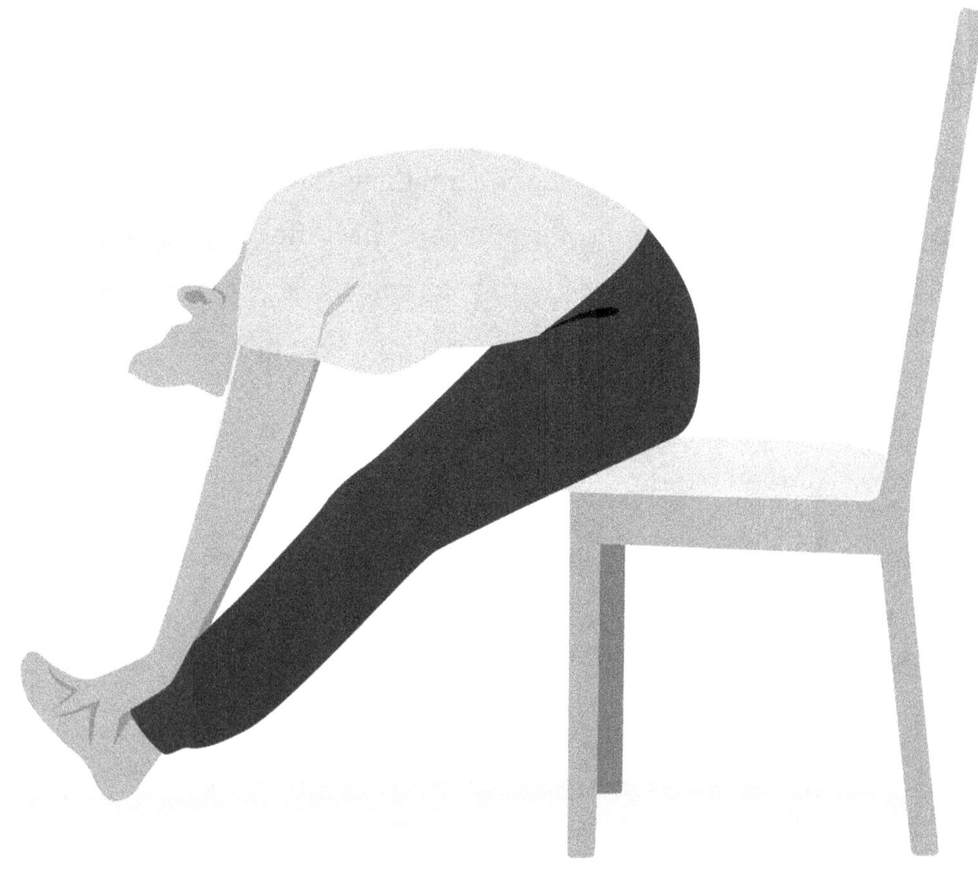

1. Start your practice by sitting upright in your chair and relaxing your neck and shoulders. Your feet should be flat on the floor, about hip-width apart, with your knees in line with your ankles. Your hands can be resting on your thighs.

2. Place your feet slightly out before you and your hands on your thighs.

3. Slowly slide your hands down your legs until you reach your feet.

4. Hold for as long as needed.

5. Slide your hands back up to your thighs.

6. Repeat.

Shoulder Pain

Chair Shoulder Stretches Help with Shoulder Pain by:

- Relieving Tension: Loosens tight shoulder muscles, reducing tension and discomfort.

- Improving Flexibility: Enhances the range of motion in the shoulder joint, decreasing stiffness.

- Promoting Circulation: Increases blood flow to the shoulder area, aiding in muscle recovery and pain relief.

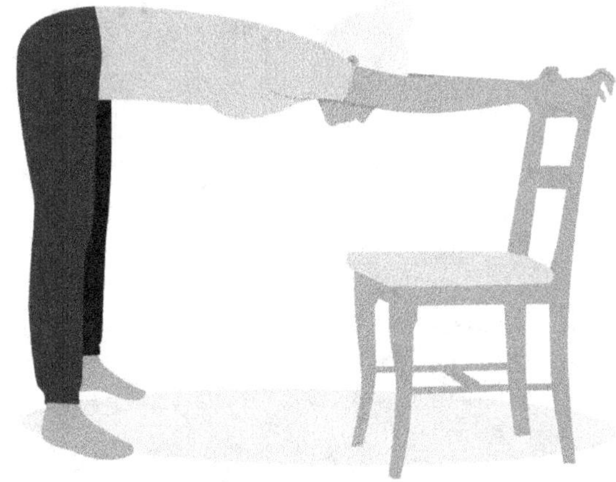

1. Begin by standing upright behind your chair. Relax your shoulders and your neck. Keep your feet about hip-width apart.

2. Take a step back from your chair and bend forward from your hips. Rest your hands on the back of the chair; they should be almost straight, with a slight bend in the elbow.

3. Lower your chest further down to feel a stretch in your shoulders and the back of your legs.

4. Hold for as long as needed.

Neck Pain

Neck Rolls Help with Neck Pain by:

- Relieving Tension: Loosens tight neck muscles, reducing stiffness and discomfort.

- Improving Flexibility: Enhances the range of motion in the neck, making it easier to move without pain.

- Promoting Circulation: Increases blood flow to the neck area, aiding in muscle relaxation and pain relief.

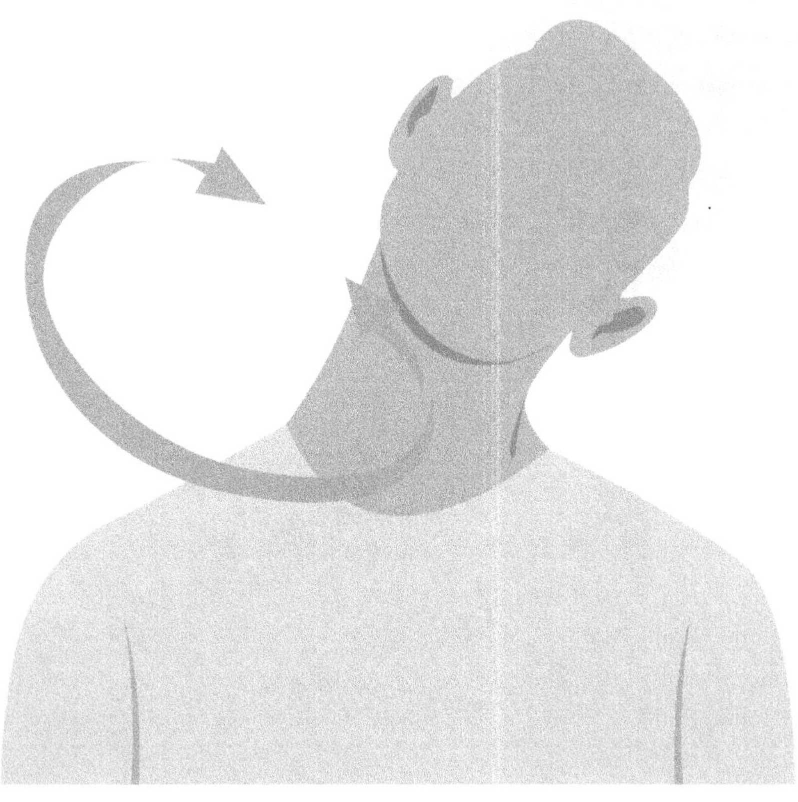

1. Start your practice by sitting upright in your chair and relaxing your neck and shoulders. Your feet should be flat on the floor, about hip-width apart, with your knees in line with your ankles. Your hands can be resting on your thighs.

2. Gently bring your right ear to your right shoulder, and rotate your head in a clockwise direction.

3. Rotate for as many repetitions as required.

4. Relax and switch directions.

Overhead Side Stretches Helps with Neck Pain by:

- Relieving Tension: Stretches the neck and upper back muscles, easing tightness and reducing discomfort.

- Improving Flexibility: Increases the neck's and shoulders' range of motion, which helps to reduce stiffness.

- Promoting Alignment: Helps maintain proper posture, which can lessen the tension on the upper back and neck.

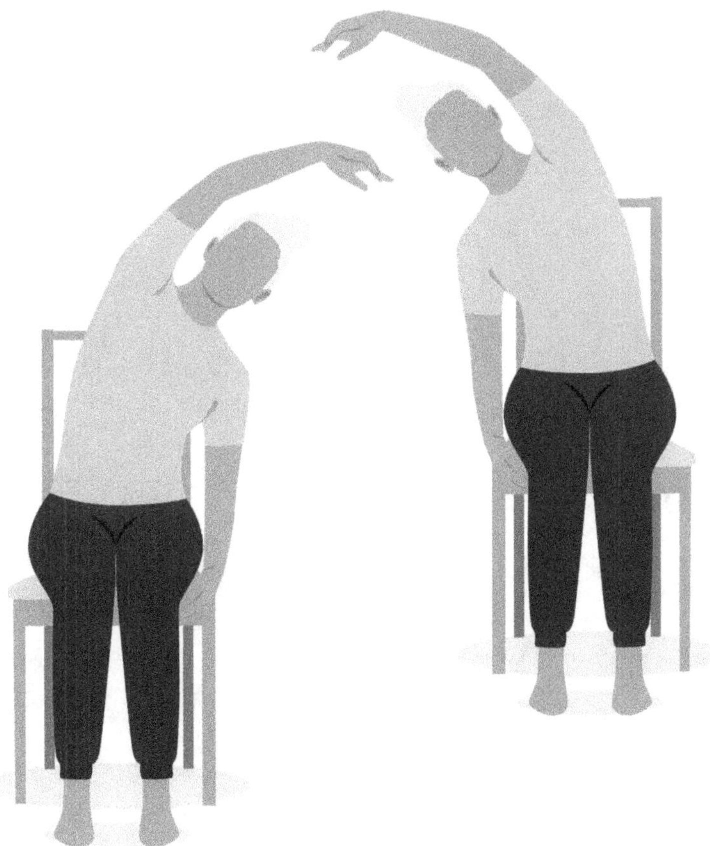

1. Start your practice by sitting upright in your chair and relaxing your neck and shoulders. Your feet should be flat on the floor, about hip-width apart, with your knees in line with your ankles. Your hands can be resting on your thighs.

2. Raise your left arm overhead, keeping it in line with your ears.

3. Reach to the right, keeping your torso facing forward.

4. Hold for 30 seconds.

5. Swap arms and repeat.

Upper Back Pain

Cat-Cow Pose Helps with Upper Back Pain by:

- Increasing Mobility: Alternating between arching and rounding the back improves flexibility and range of motion in the upper back.

- Releasing Tension: Gently stretches and relaxes the muscles in the upper back, reducing tightness and discomfort.

- Enhancing Circulation: Promotes blood flow to the spinal muscles, aiding in muscle recovery and pain relief.

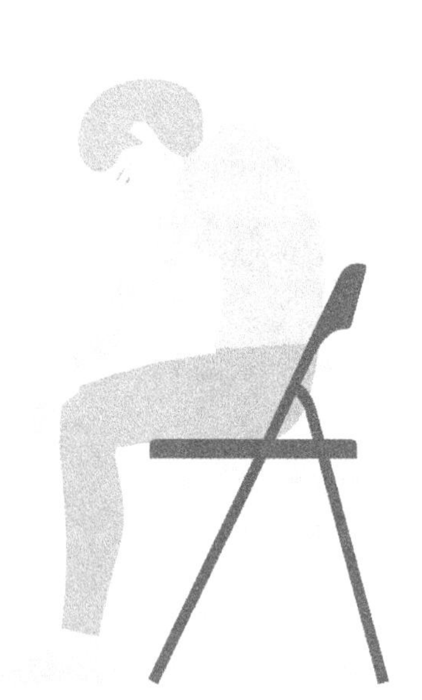 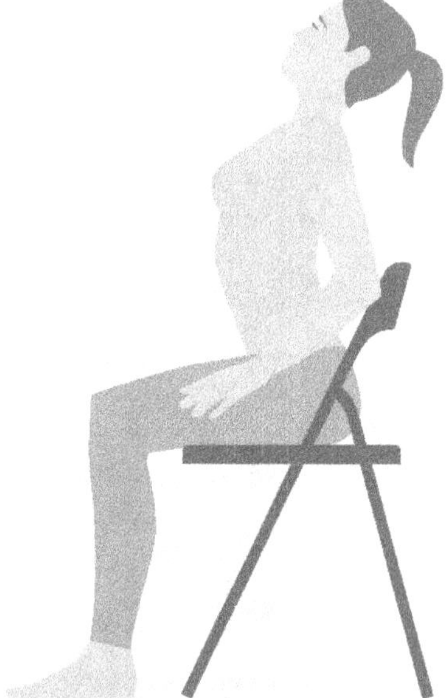

1. Start your practice by sitting upright in your chair and relaxing your neck and shoulders. Your feet should be flat on the floor, about hip-width apart, with your knees in line with your ankles. Your hands can be resting on your thighs.

2. Breathe in, round your spine, and lower your chin to your chest.

3. Breathe in and out deeply as you hold for as long as needed.

4. Breathe in and arch your back while looking up at the ceiling.

5. Breathe in and out deeply as you hold for as long as needed.

6. When you are ready to release, breathe out and slowly roll your head up to a neutral position.

Back Extensions Helps with Upper Back Pain by:

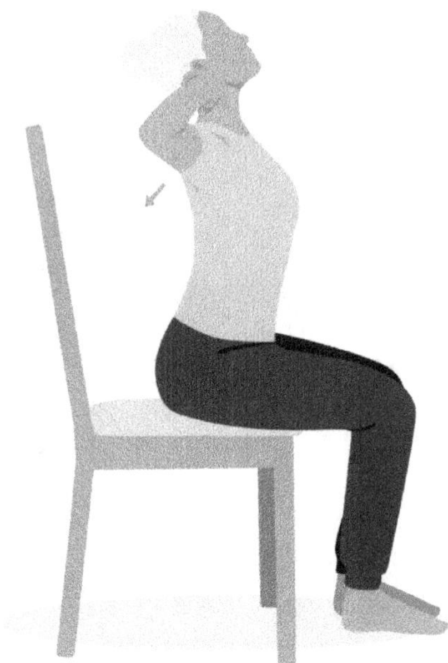

1. Start your practice by sitting upright in your chair and relaxing your neck and shoulders. Your feet should be flat on the floor, about hip-width apart, with your knees in line with your ankles. Your hands can be resting on your thighs.

2. Interlace your fingers behind your neck, with your elbows out to your sides and wide.

3. Lean back on the backrest of your chair while arching your back and pushing your chest out in front of you.

4. Hold this position for 10-15 seconds.

Sciatica

Chair Downward-Facing Dog Helps with Sciatica by:

- Stretching: The sciatic nerve can be relieved of pressure by extending the spine and stretching the hamstrings and lower back.

- Decompressing: Reduces spinal compression, helping to alleviate sciatic nerve pain.

- Improving Posture: Promotes better spinal alignment, which can help reduce sciatic discomfort.

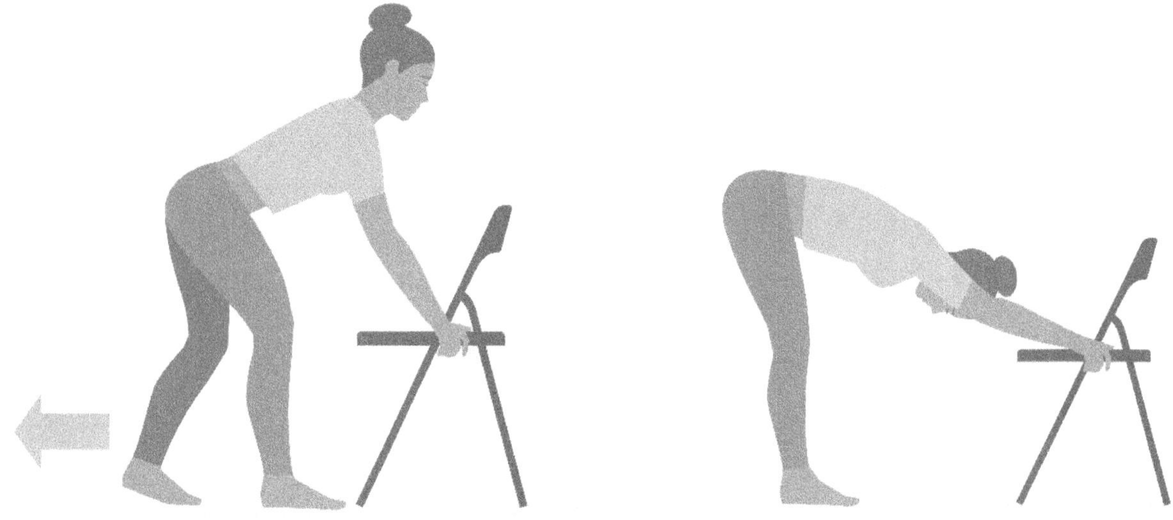

1. Start your practice by standing in front of your chair. Relax your neck and shoulders. Your feet should be hip-width apart.

2. Place your hands on the seat of your chair and carefully walk your feet backward until your body is at a 45-degree angle to the floor.

3. Breathe in and activate your midline muscles; your lower back and hips should be raised and your head and shoulders relaxed.

4. Hold this pose for as long as needed, and when you are ready to release, walk your feet back toward the chair and stand up.

Happy Baby Pose Helps with Sciatica by:

- Stretching: Deeply stretches the lower back, hips, and hamstrings, which can alleviate pressure on the sciatic nerve.

- Releasing Tension: Eases muscle tightness in the lower back and hips, reducing sciatic nerve pain.

- Improving Flexibility: Enhances the range of motion in the hips and lower back, helping to prevent sciatic flare-ups.

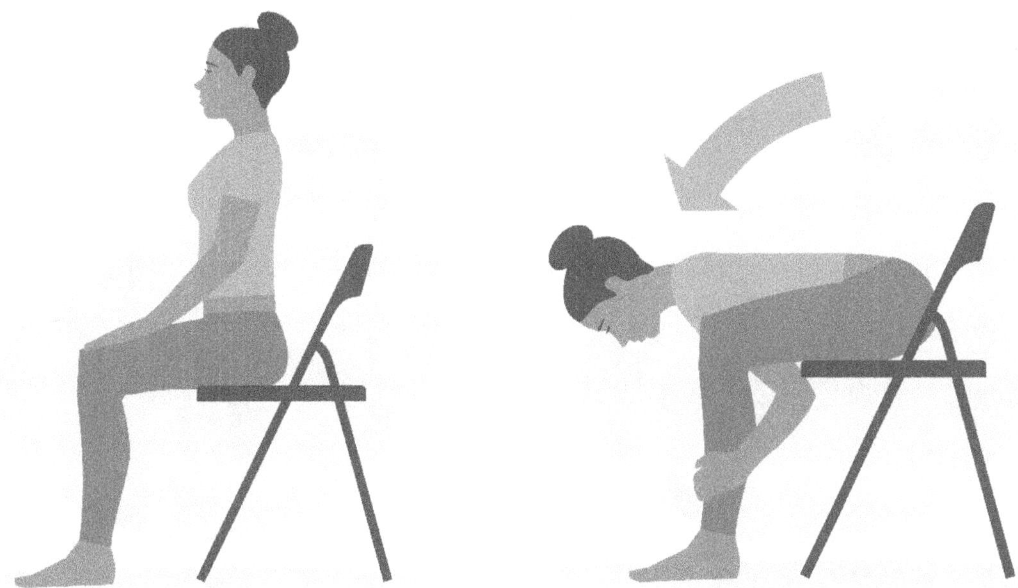

1. Start your practice by sitting upright toward the front of your chair. Relax your neck and shoulders. Your feet should be flat on the floor, a little further than hip-width apart, with your knees in line with your ankles. Your hands can be resting on your thighs.

2. Breathe in and fold forward from your waist, bringing your naval between your thighs. You may need to widen your legs to make more space for your upper body.

3. As you breathe in, reach down and take hold of your shins, ankles, or feet.

4. Carefully pull your torso down as you lower your body toward the floor.

5. Breathe in and out in this position for as long as needed.

6. When you are ready, you can release the pose by letting go of your legs and lifting your upper body back to its neutral seated position.

Arthritis-Related Pain

Identifying a single "best" yoga pose for different types of arthritis is challenging, as the effectiveness of poses can vary greatly depending on the individual and the specific joints affected. However, we can discuss some generally beneficial poses for common types of arthritis.

Osteoarthritis

For osteoarthritis, gentle stretching poses like Cat-Cow can be helpful, especially for those with spine or hip arthritis. This pose promotes flexibility and circulation in the spine without putting excessive stress on weight-bearing joints.

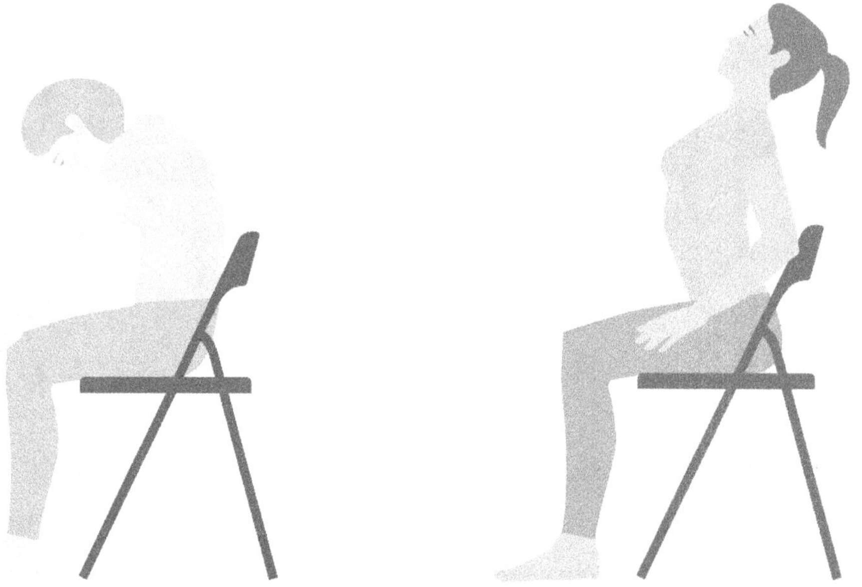

1. Start your practice by sitting upright in your chair and relaxing your neck and shoulders. Your feet should be flat on the floor, about hip-width apart, with your knees in line with your ankles. Your hands can be resting on your thighs.

2.   Breathe in, round your spine, and lower your chin to your chest.

3.   Breathe in and out deeply as you hold for as long as needed.

4.   Breathe in and arch your back while looking up at the ceiling.

5.   Breathe in and out deeply as you hold for as long as needed.

6.   When you are ready to release, breathe out and slowly roll your head up to a neutral position.

Rheumatoid Arthritis

For rheumatoid arthritis, which often affects smaller joints like those in the hands and feet, a simple Happy Baby Pose can provide gentle stretching and improved circulation to extremities.

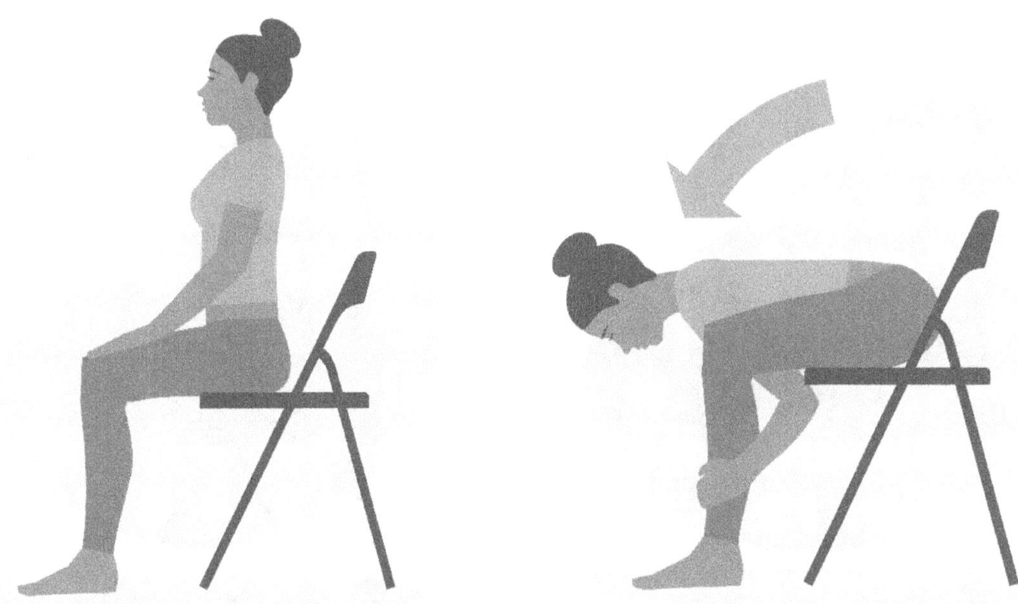

1.   Start your practice by sitting upright toward the front of your chair. Relax your neck and shoulders. Your feet should be flat on the floor, a little further than hip-width apart, with your knees in line with your ankles. Your hands can be resting on your thighs.

2.   Breathe in and fold forward from your waist, bringing your naval between your thighs. You may need to widen your legs to make more space for your upper body.

3.   As you breathe in, reach down and take hold of your shins, ankles, or feet.

4. Carefully pull your torso down as you lower your body toward the floor.

5. Breathe in and out in this position for as long as needed.

6. When you are ready, you can release the pose by letting go of your legs and lifting your upper body back to its neutral seated position.

Psoriatic Arthritis & Ankylosing Spondylitis

Those with psoriatic arthritis, which can cause both joint pain and skin irritation, may find relief in gentle twisting poses like the Seated Twist which promotes overall circulation without putting pressure on affected skin areas.

For ankylosing spondylitis, a beneficial chair yoga pose could be the Seated Twist. This pose can be performed while sitting in a chair and helps maintain spinal mobility, which is crucial for those with ankylosing spondylitis.

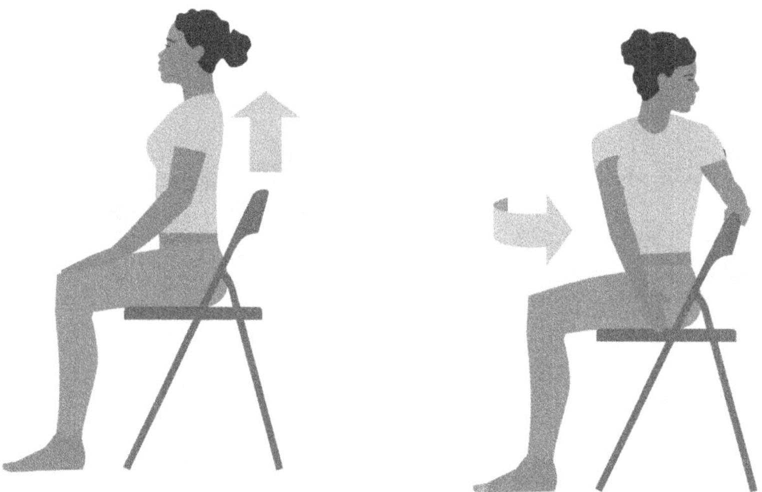

1. Start your practice by sitting upright in your chair and relaxing your neck and shoulders. Your feet should be flat on the floor, about hip-width apart, with your knees in line with your ankles. Your hands can be resting on your thighs.

2. Breathe in as you lengthen your spine, and as you breathe out, twist to the right.

3. Put your right hand on the chair's back and your left hand on the outside of your right thigh.

4. Keep your spine long and twist from your torso, not just from your shoulders.

5.   Look over your right shoulder for a deeper twist.

6.   Hold the twist for as long as needed.

7.   Inhale to release the twist back to the center.

8.   Repeat the twist on the other side by twisting to the left.

It's crucial to remember that these suggestions are general, and individuals should always consult with their healthcare provider and a qualified yoga instructor to develop a safe, personalized practice that takes into account their specific condition and limitations.

Key Takeaways

- Chair yoga is accessible to those with illnesses like osteoporosis and arthritis since it can be adjusted to meet individual needs.

- Bone health becomes increasingly crucial with age, and yoga, through its weight-bearing poses and mindfulness practices, can promote bone strength and reduce fracture risks.

- Yoga, including chair yoga, plays a significant role in managing chronic pain by addressing both physical discomfort and mental well-being.

- Yoga helps you develop a strong mental and physical connection, which enhances your ability to attend to your emotional and physical needs.

- Specific poses like the cat-cow pose, seated twist, and happy baby pose can help you alleviate chronic pain, enhance balance, and regain control over your body.

CHAPTER 7

The Joy of Movement

My goal is for you to fall in love with moving your body. I want you to experience the physical and mental benefits of movement. To be honest, I am a strong advocate for any type of movement, from Zumba to CrossFit, but it is safe to say that I am particularly fond of yoga because of the holistic benefits it brings.

We have discussed this before, so you are aware that yoga meets both our physical and mental wellness needs, but let's look into these benefits a little deeper.

Understanding the Emotional Benefits of Yoga

There are many psychological benefits to yoga:

Promoting Other Healthy Habits

If you practice yoga, you are more likely to be someone who looks after your health and well-being, which means you make choices based on maintaining wellness.

Yoga may introduce you to other like-minded individuals, and you may find yourself surrounded by people who take their health seriously and whose habits begin to influence yours.

Improving Sleep

Yoga can help increase how long you sleep as well as improve your sleep quality. Additionally, it has been shown that yoga can improve your sleep efficiency, which is the measure of how much time you spend sleeping compared to the time spent in bed (Brennan, 2021).

Improving Mental Health

Yoga can help reduce the symptoms of anxiety and depression. It is often used as an alternative form of supplementary treatment for low mood. Yoga encourages mindfulness, which helps center us while we navigate through stressful situations and periods in our lives. The breathwork that is incorporated into yoga practice is a tool that can be used off the mat to promote mental well-being.

As with other forms of exercise, yoga also encourages our body to release feel-good hormones known as endorphins. These hormones also play a role in improving and lifting our moods.

Music and Rhythm in Chair Yoga

It is well known that our brains respond favorably to music. Whether it is a soothing melody or an upbeat tempo, music can have an effect on our physiological and emotional states. Music can influence our heart rate, and motivate us to move in ways that are particular to the song. This response is not merely subjective; scientific evidence supports this claim. Studies have shown that specific rhythms can alter heart rates and induce physical responses in individuals. Music also releases dopamine, often called the "feel-good" neurotransmitter. Additionally, music also decreases the stress hormone cortisol (Beres, 2015).

Choosing the Right Music

When it comes to incorporating music into your practices, it is important to be intentional about your music selection. The tempo, lyrics, and language of music play a role in determining its impact on your activities. Choosing a high-tempo track for a mindfulness session may not be the best idea, as the fast beat may hinder your ability to unwind and engage with the present moment. Similarly, a song with lyrics can distract you and reduce your ability to stay present.

Music can really add to your practice, so I suggest that you curate a playlist for your desired mood. If you want to relax, look for ambient music characterized by gentle melodies and soothing sounds.

Key Takeaways

- Yoga has both emotional and physical benefits, such as promoting wellness-oriented decision-making and fostering connections with health-conscious communities.

- Yoga can improve sleep quality and efficiency, alleviating symptoms of anxiety and depression, and encouraging mindfulness through breathwork.

- The incorporation of music into yoga practices is supported by scientific evidence, showcasing its ability to influence heart rate, release feel-good neurotransmitters, and reduce stress hormones.

- Selecting music intentionally based on tempo, lyrics, and language is recommended to enhance the yoga experience and align with your desired mood.

CHAPTER 8

Mind-Body Harmony

This chapter is going to look at breathing exercises, guided relaxations and meditations, and mindfulness practices that can enhance your quality of life.

The Power of the Breath: Cultivating Mental Clarity and Calmness

In yoga, the breath is considered our life force, and by breathing correctly, you can enhance the benefits that you get from your practice. Prayanama refers to the yoga breath; this breathing aligns with the yoga poses and flows throughout the movements.

This intentional breathing is not confined to your yoga practice. You can practice it in day-to-day life when you need to relax and refocus yourself.

Controlled and focused breathing can increase your lung capacity, and studies have shown that it can improve the symptoms of chronic obstructive pulmonary disease (COPD). It also has great benefits for those with asthma and who are looking to improve their circulatory and respiratory function.

Deep breathing also improves your oxygen intake and helps blood move around the body more effectively. Additionally, it aids in the regulation of your autonomic nervous system, which manages bodily processes like blood pressure, digestion, and heart rate. (Omstars, n.d.).

Breathwork can also help you mentally by reducing anxiety, stress, and negative feelings and by promoting relaxation.

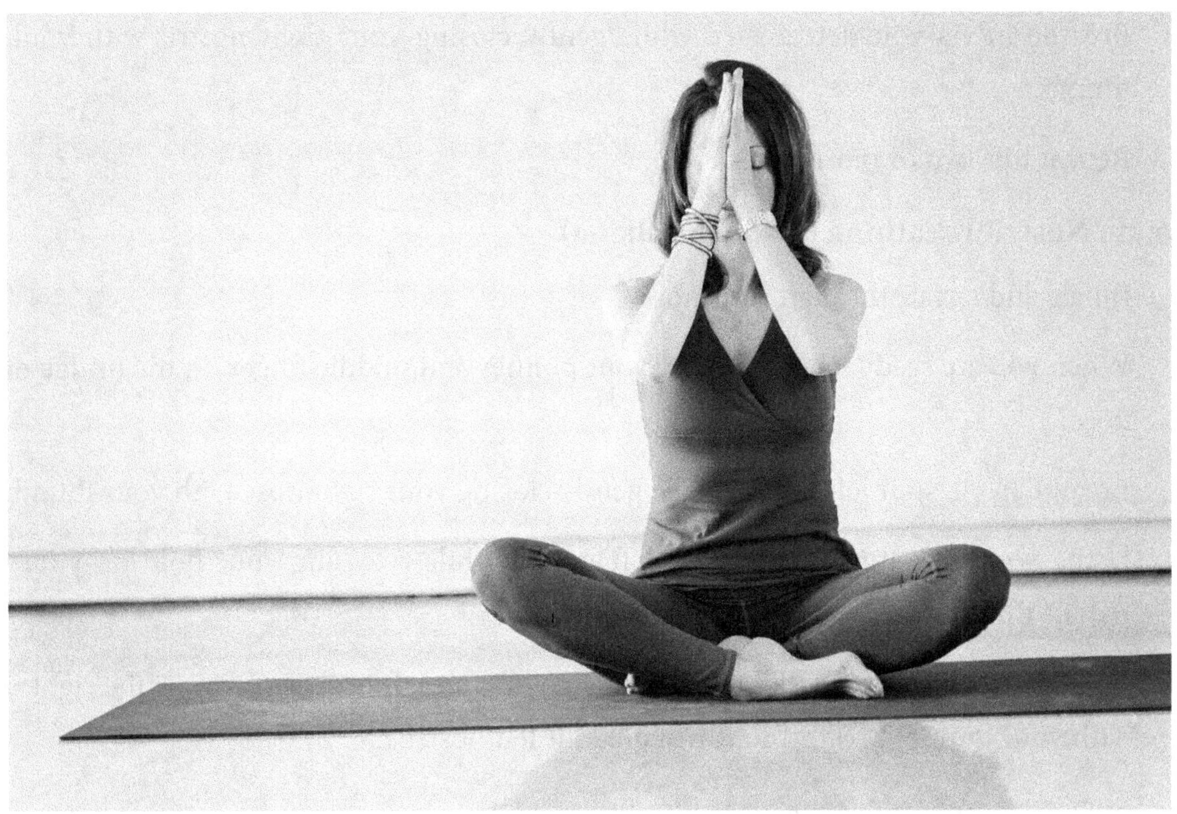

Specific Breathing Exercises for Seniors

Ocean Breath (Ujjayi)

1. Begin by taking a deep breath in through your nose, and as you breathe out, constrict the back of your throat.

2. You should make a sound that sounds very similar to the sound of waves crashing in the ocean. Alternatively, think of exhaling with an open mouth as you attempt to fog up a window or mirror.

3. Once you have learned to exhale successfully with ocean breath, you can begin to incorporate this technique with your inhales.

Lion's Breath (Simhasana)

1. You can kneel or sit on the floor or sit in a chair, depending on what feels comfortable for you. Place your hands on your knees.

2. Breathe in deeply through your nose. Exhale strongly through your mouth while you stick out your tongue. Point your tongue toward your chin and make a "haa" sound.

3. Breathe in via your left nostril while gently closing your right nostril with your right thumb.

4. Repeat this two or more times.

Alternate Nostril Breathing (Nadi Shodhana)

1. Inhale and exhale through your nose.

2. When you are ready to begin, place your pointer and middle finger on the bridge of your nose.

3. Breathe in via your left nostril while gently closing your right nose with your thumb.

4. Using your ring finger, shut your left nostril while releasing your hold on your right. Exhale through your nostril on your right.

5. Breathe in through your right nostril. Let go of your left nostril and close the right nostril with your thumb. Breathe out through your left nostril.

6. Repeat this sequence for about 10 rounds.

Three-Part Breath (Dirga Pranayama)

1. Either sit cross-legged on the floor or upright in a chair.

2. Breathe in and out through your nose, and if you feel comfortable, you can close your eyes.

3. Keep breathing through your nose, and take in a third of your full lung capacity. Focus on inhaling deep into your diaphragm and expanding your belly.

4. Breathe in the next third into your rib cage.

5. Breathe in the final third into your upper chest.

6. Breathe out through your nose in the reverse order as you release the air from your chest, then your rib cage, and then your belly.

7. Continue for 10 rounds.

Guided Relaxations

Finding Your Breath

The breath moves continually inside the body and is in constant motion. Although there is always movement, your breath is the best place to start because it's a constant you can return to anytime you need to come back to yourself.

In this relaxation, you will find your breath in your body. Return again and again to your own unique sensation of breathing.

You are training your mind to be present with one experience.

Prepare by sitting cross-legged on the floor or upright in a chair. I recommend sitting, as it helps keep the body awake and energized. Alternatively, try standing or resting flat on your back.

Let's begin.

Gently allow your eyes to close, or if you prefer to have your eyes open, you can soften your gaze and look toward the floor or the ceiling. Focus on one spot as you minimize the distractions around you.

Bring your focus to your abdomen. Relax your muscles and begin to pay attention to the rise and fall of your breath. Take a few deep breaths in and out.

Shift your focus to your chest, and as you breathe in, notice the expansion of your lungs and the rising of your chest.

As you breathe out, feel the contraction and movement.

From the beginning of the inhale until the finish of the exhale, pay attention to the flow and sensation of your breath.

Now shift your focus to your nostrils. You will find that the feeling of the breath may be more subtle.

Breathing in may cause a tiny tickle at the tip of your nose, and exhaling may make your breath appear warmer. Pick one of these three spots, your belly, chest, or nostrils, to focus on and raise your awareness.

If your thoughts wander, you can refocus by concentrating on the breath.

Stay here, focused on your breathing for a minute or two.

As you end your practice, bring this awareness with you into your daily life. To assist the mind in staying present, pay attention to your body's breathing.

Grounding

Begin by sitting cross-legged on the floor or upright in a chair. I recommend sitting, as it helps keep the body awake and energized. You can also try lying flat on your back or standing.

Gently allow your eyes to close, or if you prefer to have your eyes open, you can soften your gaze and look toward the floor or the ceiling. Focus on one spot as you minimize the distractions around you.

Breathe in fully and then breathe out slowly. Shift your focus to your breathing by noticing your breath in and your breath out, as well as the moment in between each inhalation and exhalation.

Bring your awareness to the top of your head and settle there for a moment as you notice the different sensations. Now shift your focus to your face, forehead, sides, and rear of your head.

Let your focus move to your neck before you bring awareness to your shoulders. Be mindful of the sensations you feel. Do you feel tension? Move further down to your upper arms, forearms, and finally your hands and fingers.

Move to your upper back and down your spine. Bring your attention to your chest and move toward your abdomen. Notice how your body moves as you breathe.

Shift your attention down to your lower body, moving from your thighs to your calves and shins and finally to your feet and toes.

Sense how your feet make contact with the floor. Now focus on your entire body, from your head to your feet.

Examine your entire body. Pay attention to how it feels to be seated in this particular position.

End your session with a full deep breath in and a long, slow breath out. Slowly bring your attention back to your present environment and open your eyes gently.

Move your body a bit at a time and observe how it feels. Wiggle your toes and your fingers as you continue with the rest of your day.

Key Takeaways

- Proper breathing techniques in yoga, such as Pranayama, can amplify the benefits of yoga practice and enhance overall well-being.

- Controlled and intentional breathing not only strengthens lung capacity but also aids in managing respiratory conditions like COPD and asthma.

- Breathwork plays a pivotal role in improving oxygen intake and blood circulation, and in regulating the autonomic nervous system.

- Guided relaxations like "Finding Your Breath" and "Grounding" are effective ways to improve your mindfulness, relaxation, and self-awareness.

CHAPTER 9

Beyond the Chair – Resources and Continued Learning

Should you wish to continue your learning and grow your knowledge, this chapter will provide you with websites and books about yoga and chair yoga that you can explore.

Books

- *Science Of Yoga* by Ann Swanson

- *The Eight Limbs of Yoga: A Handbook for Living Yoga Philosophy* by Stuart Ray Sarbacker and Kevin Kimple

- *Yoga: A Manual for Life* by Naomi Annand

- *The Stories Behind the Poses: Discover the Stunning Mythology Behind 50 Key Yoga Poses and Enhance Your Practice* by Raj Balkaran

- *Beyond the Mat: Don't Just Do Yoga – Live It* by Kali Om

- *The Art of Holistic Living: Yoga's Influence on Well-being And Healthy Lifestyle* by Andrew Low

- *Light on Yoga* by B. K. S. Iyengar

- *The Yoga Sutras of Patanjali* by Sri Swami Satchidananda

- *Yoga and the Quest for the True Self* by Stephen Cope

- *Yoga: The Spirit and Practice of Moving into Stillness* by Erich Schiffmann

- *Living Your Yoga: Finding the Spiritual in Everyday Life* by Judith Hanson Lasater

- *Chair Yoga for You – A Practical Guide* by Clarissa C. Adkins, Olivette Baugh Robinson, and Barbara Leaf Stewart

- *All I Need Is This Chair Yoga* by Wilma Carter

124

- *SunLight Chair Yoga – Yoga for Everyone!* by Stacie Dooreck

- *Chair Yoga for Seniors* by Lynn Lehmkuhl

Communities

- Sangha Studio – https://www.sanghastudio.org/chair-yoga-online.html

- Yin Traveller – https://www.yintraveler.com/chair-yoga-workshop

- Mind Body Online – https://www.mindbodyonline.com/explore/fitness/classes-online/livestream-chair-yoga-community-class-yoga-house-llc-northeast-los-angeles

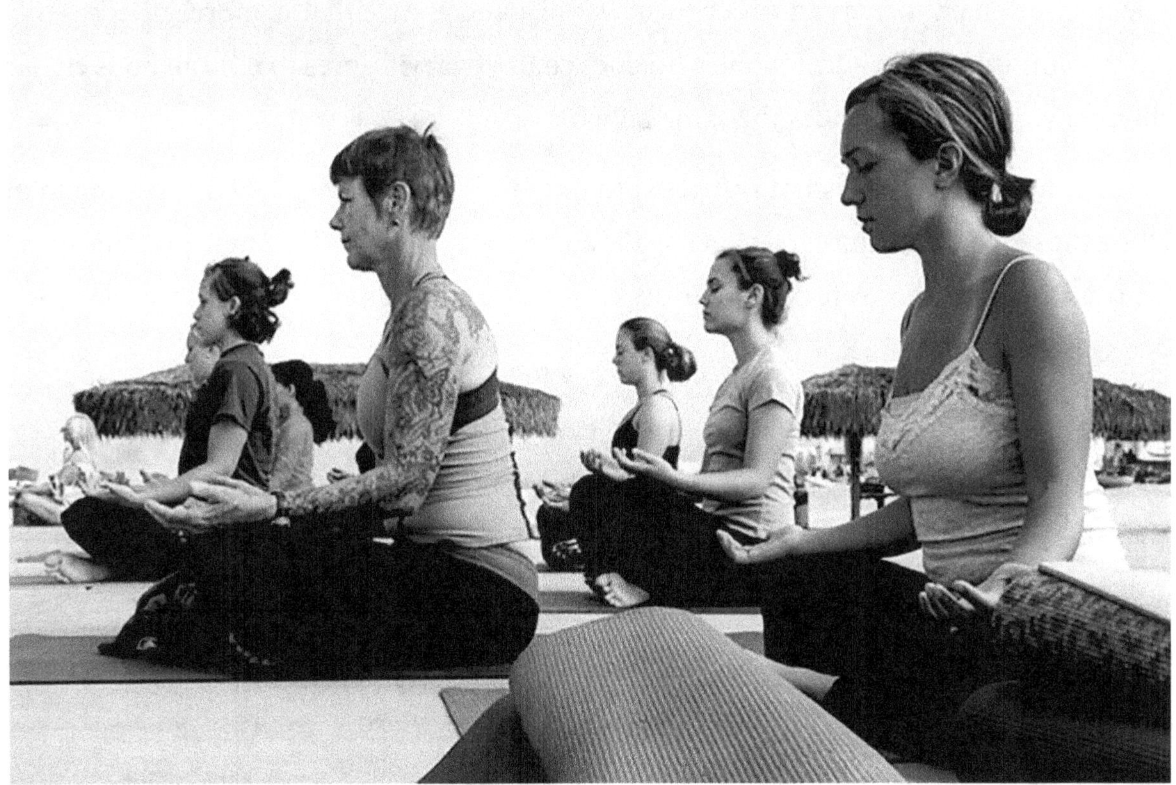

CHAPTER 10

Common Questions and Practical Tips

Common Misconceptions About Chair Yoga

Chair Yoga Is Only for Seniors

Many people see chair yoga as an easier form of yoga and a style that is more suited to the older population. This is not true, and anyone who does chair yoga will agree that it can be as challenging as traditional yoga and it provides the same benefits.

Chair yoga is for anyone and is not restricted to only those who have problems getting in and off the mat or those who are injured. Chair yoga is a great way to introduce new practitioners to the exercise It is useful for those stuck at their desks but who still want to move, as well as those short on space and time.

It Is Just Seated Stretching

Chair yoga takes traditional yoga poses and adapts them for the use of a chair, and there are many ways that these poses can be modified, either by sitting on the chair or by using it as a prop.

The chair yoga poses target the same muscle groups as the traditional poses, and of course, the practice also incorporates mindfulness and breathwork. Static and dynamic holds and flows are used, and these are held for short or long periods of time.

You will find that you can adapt any of your favorite flows, and you are not limited to purely static stretches.

It Is Too Easy

This is a common misconception. Chair yoga is not an easier version of yoga; it is a modified version. If done correctly, it will be able to give you the same challenge as a traditional yoga class.

You Need a Special Chair

As with all yoga, you do not need fancy, specific equipment. In this case, all you need is a suitable chair; in most cases, you will already have one at home. Almost any chair will work, but your best options are ones with a straight back, a wide enough chair seat, no armrests, and a height that allows your knees to bend at 90 degrees while your feet stay on the floor.

Common Problems

Sometimes you just need simple tweaks here and there to fix a practice that has gotten old or poses and postures that do not feel right. Here are some common things to tick off if you are feeling like your practice is lacking and to help boost your flows.

- Find a good chair and ideally choose one that you love.

- Always keep your feet flat on the floor when you practice, unless your pose demands otherwise. This helps keep you grounded.

- Take your time and go slowly.

- Practice your breathwork and focus on your breath throughout your flow.

- Add music to your practice, as this adds another sensory experience.

Staying Motivated

Practicing yoga from home has both positive and negative aspects when it comes to motivation and accountability. You can argue both sides with valid reasons for each point. For example, practicing yoga from home is better because it is easy to walk to your yoga space and do your practice. You do not need to travel or take too much time out of your day. It is very convenient.

On the other hand, classes are more social and you become a part of a community. You are also held more accountable and find it more motivating to attend a class than to have to work out at home by yourself.

A common problem when practicing from home is procrastination; this will impact our ability to create a routine. Again, this boils down to motivation and getting yourself dressed and on your chair to practice. Without an accountability partner or support system, this becomes difficult.

Try to schedule your sessions in your diary and treat them as an important meeting with yourself. You can schedule them at the same time each day to make it easier to fall into a routine. You can also set up your mat and chair the night before so that your space is ready for you, and all you need to do is sit down and begin.

Alternatively, set up your own dedicated yoga space for yourself. We discussed this in Chapter 2, where we determined that you do not need a lot of space but having an inviting space makes it more likely for you to maintain a consistent practice.

Finally, track your progress. Whether your clothes fit better, you are more flexible, or you can hold a pose for longer than you used to be able to—these are small milestones that should be recognized and celebrated. They remind you how far you have come and that you are making progress toward your goals.

Speaking of goals, make sure that they are small and attainable while still being fairly challenging. Take your bigger goal and break it down into smaller ones, as this will keep you motivated and moving forward.

Frequently Asked Questions

I have never done yoga before. Can I do chair yoga?

Of course! Chair yoga is a great introduction to traditional yoga and can be customized to your individual needs. You can adapt it to be more basic or more challenging, depending on your experience and fitness levels.

Do I need specific clothes?

No, you do not need any special clothes for yoga. All you need is something comfortable that you can move in. You will want to avoid wearing clothes that have buttons or zippers, which may be uncomfortable. You can also practice barefoot or in socks that also have a grip on the sole.

Do I need a special chair?

Some chairs are made specifically for chair yoga, but they are not required. You can make do with a kitchen chair, stool, or even a desk chair.

Make sure that the chair you use is safe and sturdy and will not slip on your floor.

I have joint issues. Could chair yoga aggravate them?

You should always get the all-clear from your healthcare provider before beginning any kind of exercise. Chat with your healthcare provider, and should there be any issues, they can advise accordingly.

What are some of the most common poses?

Some of the more common poses are cat-cow, side bends, forward fold, seated twist, downward dog, and eagle arms.

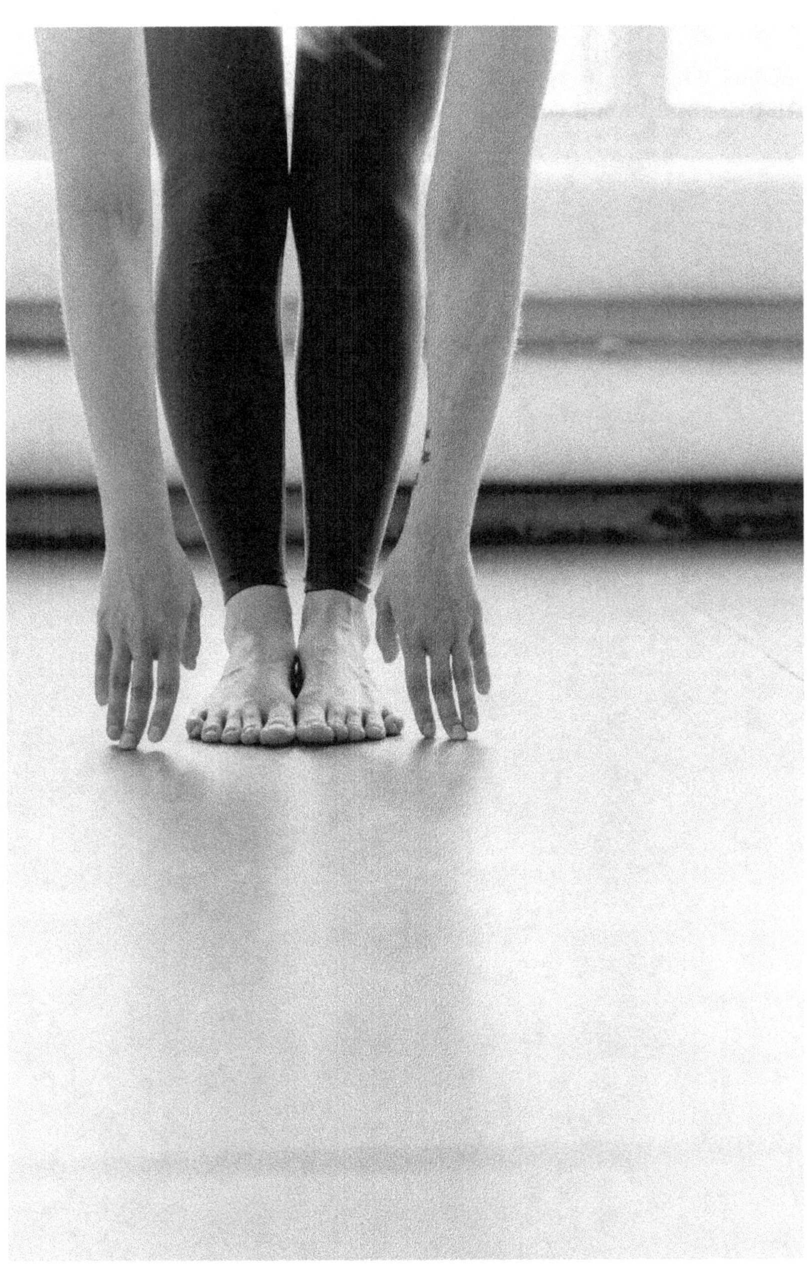

Key Takeaways

- Chair yoga is not limited to seniors and can provide similar challenges and benefits as traditional yoga for practitioners of all ages.

- Chair yoga involves modified poses targeting the same muscle groups as traditional yoga, incorporating mindfulness, breathwork, and various hold durations.

- Basic chairs with specific features like a straight back and appropriate height are sufficient for chair yoga practice.

- Beginners can participate in chair yoga as an introduction to traditional yoga, with poses that can be customized based on individual needs and fitness levels.

Conclusion

You are now set to continue your yoga journey.

Through gentle movements, mindful breathing techniques, and relaxation practices, chair yoga can support your physical rehabilitation, weight loss, and flexibility. It can help you become more mentally clear, straighten your posture, and lessen stiffness in your joints. It can even serve as an alternative treatment for chronic pain.

We do not need to worry about aging and getting older if we are smart about our health and wellness. As we get older, we are told that we are going to lose independence, strength and mental abilities, and a range of other negative narratives get thrown our way, but it does not need to be like this.

This book gives you tools that will help you age gracefully without losing your independence and ensure that you continue to do the things you love and lead a life full of vibrancy and vitality.

<h1 style="text-align:center">References</h1>

10 tips to help you make exercise a habit. (n.d.). Www.carecredit.com. Retrieved May 21, 2024, from https://www.carecredit.com/well-u/health-wellness/how-to-make-exercise-a-habit/

Beres , D. (2015, April 1). *Why music in yoga matters.* Teach.yoga. https://teach.yoga/why-music-in-yoga-matters/

Brennan, D. (2021, October 25). *Benefits of yoga for mental health.* WebMD. https://www.webmd.com/balance/benefits-of-yoga-for-mental-health

Burger, T. (2020, June 1). *50 yoga quotes: Best, happy, inspiring & motivational.* TeganBYoga New. https://www.teganbyoga.com/post/best-yoga-quotes

Calm. (n.d.). 6 benefits of yoga for mental health (and how to practice) — Calm Blog. *Calm Blog.* https://www.calm.com/blog/benefits-of-yoga-for-mental-health

CDC. (2023, October 31). *Adults need more physical activity.* Centers for Disease Control and Prevention. https://www.cdc.gov/physicalactivity/inactivity-among-adults-50plus

Clear, J. (2014, September 19). *3 simple ways to make exercise a habit.* James Clear. https://jamesclear.com/exercise-habit

Davis, N. (2021, August 30). *Resistance and mobility training are key for healthy aging.* Healthline. https://www.healthline.com/health/fitness/healthy-aging-guide-to-strength-training

Doran Yoga. (2020, June 24). *Yoga for seniors, sun salutation on a chair. suitable for most.* Doron Yoga. https://doronyoga.com/yoga-for-seniors-sun-salutation-on-a-chair/

Drake, K. (2022, June 22). *What is chair yoga? What are its benefits?* GoodRx. https://www.goodrx.com/well-being/movement-exercise/chair-yoga

Elaine Oyang. (2021, October 19). *3 minute gentle chair yoga for chronic pain.* YouTube. https://www.youtube.com/watch?v=294XqPsjzr8

Flowwithme. (2021, February 9). *What chair is good for chair yoga?* Flowithme. https://www.flowithme.com/post/what-chair-is-good-for-chair-yoga

Healthline. (2017, March 1). *The ultimate "deskercise" routine: Stretches for the office.* Healthline. https://www.healthline.com/health/deskercise#1

History of yoga: Origins to modern day | origym. (2022, March 8). Origympersonaltrainercourses.co.uk. https://origympersonaltrainercourses.co.uk/blog/history-of-yoga

Jeffries, T. (2022, July 3). *13 chair yoga poses you can do without leaving your seat.* Yoga Journal. https://www.yogajournal.com/yoga-101/types-of-yoga/chair-yoga-poses/

Jeraci, A. R. (n.d.). *Chair yoga flow: A dynamic way to sit and practice.* Yogainternational.com. Retrieved May 15, 2024, from https://yogainternational.com/article/view/chair-yoga-flow-a-dynamic-way-to-sit-and-practice/

Johns Hopkins Rheumatology. (2019, June 26). *Yoga for arthritis : Chair yoga for improved mobility : Johns Hopkins Arthritis Center.* Www.youtube.com. https://www.youtube.com/watch?v=yUnZzpX2KMw

Kinshipe Pointe. (2021, December 9). *Why flexibility is important for seniors.* Kinship Pointe. https://kinshippointe.com/why-flexibility-is-important-for-seniors/

Lee, A. (2022, July 5). *The ultimate yoga teacher's guide for creating yoga sequences.* Beyogi. https://beyogi.com/the-ultimate-guide-for-creating-yoga-sequences/

Madhivanan, P., Krupp, K., Waechter, R., & Shidhaye, R. (2021). Yoga for Healthy Aging: Science or Hype? *Advances in Geriatric Medicine and Research, 3*(3). https://doi.org/10.20900/agmr20210016

Masterclass. (2021, July 7). *Yoga props guide: 8 types of props for practicing yoga.* Masterclass. https://www.masterclass.com/articles/yoga-props-guide

Metro Physical Therapy. (2020, July 4). *Metro Chair Yoga - "Freedom Flow."* Www.youtube.com. https://youtu.be/CJej-Hz9Xf4?si=diCtgEvzSP9bW40R

Miranda, S. (2023, July 21). *How to mentally prepare for your yoga retreat: Tips and tricks.* Yoga Lounge Portugal. https://yogalounge.pt/prepare-for-your-yoga-retreat/

Mobley, T. (2017, August 24). *Why everyone should adopt A yogi's mindset.* Taylor, Lately. https://taylorlately.com/everyone-adopt-yogis-mindset

More Life Health. (n.d.). *Exercise library for seniors* . More Life Health - Seniors Health & Fitness. https://morelifehealth.com/exercise-library

Nash, J. (2022, June 19). *How to practice visualization meditation: 3 best scripts.* PositivePsychology.com. https://positivepsychology.com/visualization-meditation/#scripts

Omstars. (n.d.). *Breathing for yoga: Why its important and how to do it right – omstars.* Omstars.com. https://omstars.com/blog/practice/breathing-for-yoga-why-its-important-and-how-to-do-it-right/

Perkins, T. (2023, February 8). *Chair yoga myths.* Trin Perkins, M.S.Ed | Corporate Yoga Instructor. https://trinperkins.com/chair-yoga-myths/

Precision Nutrition . (n.d.). *Worksheet: The 5 Whys For clients.* https://assets.precisionnutrition.com/2019/08/worksheet-the-5-whys.pdf

Pureful Yoga Team. (2022, February 11). *The history of yoga - A timeline from inception to present day.* Pureful Yoga. https://purefulyoga.com/blog/history-of-yoga/

Rusack, P. (2023, March 22). *70+ growth mindset quotes about hard work and perseverance.* We Are Teachers. https://www.weareteachers.com/growth-mindset-quotes/

Sattva Yoga Academy. (n.d.). *The importance of alignment and posture in yoga | tips for proper technique.* Sattvayogaacademy.com. Retrieved May 13, 2024, from https://sattvayogaacademy.com/importance-alignment-and-posture-yoga

SeniorShape Fitness. (2022, March 14). *Chair yoga stretch & strength // seated exercises for seniors & beginners.* Www.youtube.com. https://youtu.be/gXB3NhOAalk?si=eYSiA4lDGpvHS4SR

SeniorShape Fitness. (2022b, June 27). *Stretching exercises for beginners & seniors // standing & seated workout for flexibility & mobility.* YouTube. https://www.youtube.com/watch?v=3cSmYMYOciI

Sullivan Barger, T. (2022, March 22). *Yoga for osteoporosis in the spine.* Www.healthcentral.com. https://www.healthcentral.com/condition/osteoporosis/yoga-osteoporosis

Taking Charge. (n.d.). *Guided imagery script.*
https://www.takingcharge.csh.umn.edu/survivorship/sites/default/files/PDFs/Guided%20Im
agery%20Script.pdf

WebMD. (2019). *Slideshow: 12 basic yoga poses.* WebMD. https://www.webmd.com/fitness-
exercise/ss/slideshow-yoga-pose-basics

Williams, C. (2023, January 27). *A beginner's guide to yoga props: 4 essential yoga props.*
YogaRenew. https://www.yogarenewteachertraining.com/a-beginners-guide-to-yoga-props-
4-essential-yoga-props/

Yes2next. (2022, June 14). *Chair yoga for seniors, beginners.* Www.youtube.com.
https://youtu.be/U_jdXFfegKE?si=uvwjceWkidcOgtuU

YJ Editors. (2017, April 13). *Warrior I pose (virabhadrasana I).* Yoga Journal.
https://www.yogajournal.com/poses/warrior-i-pose/

Yoga by Kierstie Payge. (2023, February 5). *Chair yoga for core strength - for seniors.* YouTube.
https://www.youtube.com/watch?v=Dmu7L0jBvKs

Yoga With Adriene. (2017, July 23). *Chair yoga - yoga for seniors | Yoga with Adriene.*
Www.youtube.com. https://youtu.be/-Ts01MC2mIo?si=gCa26hkBzgK_1yBm

Yoga with Joelle. (2021, June 21). *Chair yoga for fibromyalgia and chronic pain - gentle seated
stretches.* YouTube. https://www.youtube.com/watch?v=nMw_DtRtSJc

Yoga with Kassandra. (2019, July 11). *Gentle chair yoga for beginners and seniors.*
Www.youtube.com. https://youtu.be/1DYH5ud3zHo?si=IVqWpS0_wWIk403G

Yoganama. (2021, January 13). *Balance exercises for seniors | level 3.* YouTube.
https://www.youtube.com/watch?v=aKvA3GwmjPU&t=46s

Images

Caballero, M. (2020). Woman-in-white-tank-top-and-black-shorts-sitting-on-brown-wooden-floor [Image]. In *https://unsplash.com/*. https://unsplash.com/photos/woman-in-white-tank-top-and-black-shorts-sitting-on-brown-wooden-floor-LRcPNV8HQ3Q

EnergieDeVie. (2019). Yoga-meditation-pose-meditate-4489430 [Image]. In *https://pixabay.com/*. https://pixabay.com/photos/yoga-meditation-pose-meditate-4489430/

Janeb13. (2016). Women-yoga-class-fitness-asana-1179435/ [Image]. In *https://pixabay.com/*. https://unsplash.com/s/photos/yoga-classes?license=free

laurajuarez. (2019). Yoga-meditation-fitness-mindfulness-4595164 [Image]. In *https://pixabay.com/*. https://pixabay.com/photos/yoga-meditation-fitness-mindfulness-4595164/

Lavern, M. (2011). Woman-stretching-wearing-black-bra-and-pants-D2uK7elFBU4 [Image]. In *https://unsplash.com/*. https://unsplash.com/photos/woman-stretching-wearing-black-bra-and-pants-D2uK7elFBU4

May, K. (2020). Woman-in-black-shirt-and-gray-pants-sitting-on-brown-wooden-bench-6CLBoiWuzSU [Image]. In *https://unsplash.com/*. https://unsplash.com/photos/woman-in-black-shirt-and-gray-pants-sitting-on-brown-wooden-bench-6CLBoiWuzSU

Northe, C. (2016). Yoga-exercise-sports-fitness [Image]. In *https://pixabay.com/*. https://unsplash.com/s/photos/chair-yoga?license=free

OPPO Find X5 Pro. (2022). A-person-sitting-on-a-beach [Image]. In *https://unsplash.com/*. https://unsplash.com/photos/a-person-sitting-on-a-beach-fNPsd6_ZiuA

photo-graphe. (2016). Yoga, zen, fitness image [Image]. In *https://pixabay.com/*. https://pixabay.com/photos/yoga-zen-fitness-practice-yoga-1714757/

Rubo, A. (2022). A-pair-of-legs-and-feet [Image]. In *https://unsplash.com/*. https://unsplash.com/photos/a-pair-of-legs-and-feet-SYX4S7SVBOM

The Nix Company. (2020). Black-and-white-speakers-on-white-shelf [Image]. In *https://unsplash.com.* https://unsplash.com/photos/black-and-white-speakers-on-white-shelf-biX8sBfNcPc

Wetton, D. (2019). Woman-performing-yoga-t1NEMSm1rgI [Image]. In *https://unsplash.com/*. https://unsplash.com/photos/woman-performing-yoga-t1NEMSm1rgI

Windows. (2021). A-man-doing-yoga-in-a-living-room [Image]. In https://unsplash.com/ . https://unsplash.com/photos/a-man-doing-yoga-in-a-living-room-ZQ-3NFtNOOc